Bounding Biomedicine

Bounding Biomedicine

Evidence and Rhetoric in the New Science of
Alternative Medicine

COLLEEN DERKATCH

The University of Chicago Press
Chicago and London

Colleen Derkatch is assistant professor of rhetoric in the Department of English and vice chair of the Research Ethics Board at Ryerson University in Toronto, Canada.

The University of Chicago Press, Chicago 60637
The University of Chicago Press, Ltd., London
© 2016 by The University of Chicago
All rights reserved. Published 2016.
Printed in the United States of America

25 24 23 22 21 20 19 18 17 16   1 2 3 4 5

ISBN-13: 978-0-226-34584-0 (cloth)
ISBN-13: 978-0-226-34598-7 (e-book)
DOI: 10.7208/chicago/9780226345987.001.0001

Library of Congress Cataloging-in-Publication Data

Derkatch, Colleen, author.
  Bounding biomedicine : evidence and rhetoric in the new science of alternative medicine / Colleen Derkatch.
     pages ; cm
  Includes bibliographical references and index.
  ISBN 978-0-226-34584-0 (cloth : alk. paper)—ISBN 978-0-226-34598-7 (e-book)
1. Alternative medicine—United States—History—20th century. 2. Alternative medicine—Research—United States—History—20th century. 3. Medicine—United States—History—20th century.   I. Title.
  R733.D4393 2016
  610.28—dc23

                                                    2015029053

♾ This paper meets the requirements of ANSI/NISO Z39.48-1992 (Permanence of Paper).

For Isla and Nathan,
"just for."

"[I]f you who are reading this article do not know what rational thinking means, you are beyond help."

RUDOLPH HAPPLE, "The Essence of Alternative Medicine: A Dermatologist's View from Germany"

"[Q]uackery never prospers, for if and when it does, it becomes termed medicine instead."

ROY PORTER, *Quacks: Fakers and Charlatans in English Medicine*

Contents

Acknowledgments

The basic argument of this book, that the notion of evidence is mobilized rhetorically in debates about complementary and alternative medicine, rests on the premise from science and technology studies and related fields that science both produces and is produced by communities of scholars. This is also true beyond science, of course: community is integral to any area of academic inquiry, and I am lucky and grateful to have worked with, learned from, and leaned on a great number of individuals and institutions that have formed my own community over the course of writing this book. With deepest appreciation, I acknowledge them here.

I am grateful for the financial and other assistance I received over the course of my research for this book. Early on, I received a fellowship from the Social Sciences and Humanities Research Council of Canada and, later, I received generous funding from the University of British Columbia and Ryerson University. I also thank Brooke Ballantyne, for her assistance with the journals I was writing about; James McCormack, for expecting me to understand scientific methodology as well as a scientist would; and George Lundberg, for his lively and generous reflections on his time at the *Journal of the American Medical Association*. Most importantly, I would like to thank my interview participants, who I cannot name but without whom this study would be another thing entirely.

I have presented on this research at various scholarly gatherings over the years, including conferences of the American Society for Bioethics and Humanities, the Association for the Rhetoric of Science and Technology, the Association of Teachers of Technical Writing, the Canadian Association for the Study of Discourse and Writing, the Canadian Society for the Study of Rhetoric, the National Communication Association, the Rhetoric Society of

America, and the Society for Social Studies of Science. I thank all of my co-panelists and attendees for their valuable questions and feedback. I am also grateful to the participants and attendees at the Rhetoric and Knowledge-Making in Health and Medicine workshop at the Peter Wall Institute for Advanced Studies at the University of British Columbia, and to Judy Segal for inviting me to take part. And finally, I workshopped this project in its earliest stages at the first Rhetoric Society of America Summer Institute, in a workshop on rhetoric of health and medicine, and want to acknowledge and thank all of the participants in the workshop, as well as the organizers Ellen Barton and Susan Wells.

For their assistance in preparing and revising the manuscript, I am grateful to my two anonymous peer reviewers for their helpful commentary, and to David Morrow and everyone else at the University of Chicago Press for shepherding this project so carefully and well. I also acknowledge and thank my stunningly good research assistants Shaun Pett and Julie Morrissy, who helped me manage the manuscript in the final stages and helped me keep everything else afloat in the process.

My greatest intellectual debt is to Judy Segal, once my doctoral supervisor and now colleague and friend, whom I thank for her rigor, guidance, and support, and for her fabulous companionship in many conference cities over the years. I also thank my first mentors in rhetoric and language studies, Leah Ceccarelli, Jessica de Villiers, Janet Giltrow, Herbert Simons, and especially Philippa Spoel, who has since become my coresearcher and dear friend. And for taking me as a colleague when I was too junior to know much of anything, and for mentoring me so graciously since then, I thank Deborah Dysart-Gale, Joan Leach, Blake Scott, and, especially, Lisa Keränen and Amy Koerber. Beyond my own discipline, I thank Patsy Badir and Alan Richardson.

I am grateful to my former colleagues in Arts Studies in Research and Writing at the University of British Columbia and to my new colleagues in English at Ryerson. Special thanks go to my friends with whom I grew up intellectually: Mono Brown, Eddy Kent, Elizabeth Maurer, Kate Stanley, Tyson Stotle, Katja Thieme, and Terri Tomsky, as well as Julia Fawcett, Laura Fisher, and Monique Tschofen. Special thanks go to Jennifer Burwell, who read and responded to several chapters with ridiculously quick turnaround times and smart commentary.

Finally, I can only inadequately express my gratitude to those much closer to home. I thank Wynn Deschner, Kim Duff, and Heather Latimer for their stalwart friendship, support, love, kindness, and excellent taste in scotch. And to my parents, Dorothy Berg-Derkatch and Jim Derkatch, I am grateful for their constant encouragement and support, their good humor, and most of all, their patience. My hugest and happiest debts are to my daughter Isla Whitford, who has grown up alongside (and in spite of) this project and who is such a bright light and so much fun, and to Nathan Whitford, who carried so much of the load, for so long, and who gave me space and time to work (and reminded me, often, when not to).

Portions of this text have been previously published in standalone articles, although they appear here in substantially revised and expanded form, often as single paragraphs across different chapters. Chapters 1, 2, and 3 include elements of my analysis previously published in "Method as Argument: Boundary Work in Evidence-Based Medicine" (*Social Epistemology* 23.4 [2008]: 371–88), which appear here courtesy of Taylor & Francis. Chapter 2 develops arguments first published in "Demarcating Medicine's Boundaries: Constituting and Categorizing in the Journals of the American Medical Association" (*Technical Communication Quarterly* 21.3 [2012]: 210–29), also courtesy of Taylor & Francis. Chapter 4 extends my analysis first published in "Does Biomedicine Control for Rhetoric? Configuring Practitioner-Patient Interaction" (*Rhetorical Questions of Health and Medicine*, eds. Joan Leach and Deborah Dysart-Gale [Lanham, MD: Lexington Books, 2010], 129–53), with permission of Lexington Books. Finally, arguments that I develop about the notion of wellness toward the end of chapter 4 and in the conclusion emerged out of my article "'Wellness' as Incipient Illness: Dietary Supplement Discourse in a Biomedical Culture" (*Present Tense: A Journal of Rhetoric in Society* 2.2 [2012]: n.p.), which was published under a Creative Commons license.

This book tells the story of a specific moment in the history of the medical profession, one that occurred in the United States in the late twentieth century, at a time when the health care marketplace appeared to have been blown wide open by consumer demand. This historical moment in turn tells a much larger story, one that lays bare the discursive means through which some health practices and professions come to and maintain ascendancy over others. During the 1990s, unprecedented numbers of Americans turned to complementary and alternative medicine (CAM), an umbrella term encompassing a disparate range of health practices such as chiropractic, energy healing, herbal medicine, homeopathy, meditation, naturopathy, and traditional Chinese medicine. By 1997, nearly half the US population was seeking CAM, spending at least $27 billion out-of-pocket annually on related products and services (Eisenberg et al., "Trends"). As CAM rose in popularity over the decade, so did interest in mainstream medicine toward understanding whether or not those practices actually worked and, if so, how. Considerable federal research infrastructure was dedicated to testing CAM interventions in clinical trials, and medical educators scrambled to assist physicians in advising patients about CAM. This book examines how the medical profession maintained its position of privilege and prestige throughout this process, even as its foothold at the top of the health care hierarchy appeared to be crumbling.

Examining the rhetorical, persuasive dimensions of this historical moment in the medical profession captures a much larger field of vision than one might expect. As the chapters that follow reveal, the question of how to test health practices that do not fit easily (or at all) within standard frameworks of medical research is a question that sweeps us both deep into the realm of medical knowledge-making—the research teams, clinical trials, and medical journals that determine which treatments are safe and effective—and out into the world where doctors meet patients, illnesses find treatment, and values, priorities, policies, and practices collide. We see, for example, how narratives of medicine's entanglements with competing models of health care imprint much more than the historical episodes they narrate: these narratives imprint the fabric of medical knowledge itself.

We see also how the medical profession is made and remade through its own discursive activity, through the many texts that shape the working lives of medical researchers and practitioners. These texts, written and spoken, include original published research, editorials and letters in medical journals, conversations with patients about their health and treatment, and the stories that circulate in public about the work that medical professionals perform and the individuals whose lives they so profoundly affect. All of these texts have a hand in shaping the boundaries of the medical profession; this book examines one such set of texts to show how they do it. Because the line between mainstream medicine and its "alternatives" is drawn again and again over time, understanding the factors that determine its position at any one moment illuminates the rhetoricity of medicine itself.

CAM Enters Biomedicine

Prior to the 1990s, the medical profession had largely been ambivalent about complementary and alternative medicine. Individually, practitioners were often indifferent to or even supportive of CAM, provided that it did not interfere with their daily practice of medicine. As a collective entity, however, the medical profession had long engaged in efforts to protect itself against competition by adopting measures aimed at restricting alternative practitioners' rights to practice. Still, it was not until Americans' astonishingly high levels of CAM use came to light with a landmark survey published in 1993 in the *New England Journal of Medicine* that the medical profession as a whole recognized CAM as worthy of serious, sustained scientific inquiry. That survey, led by David Eisenberg at Harvard Medical School, defined as "alternative" those "medical interventions not taught widely at US medical schools or generally available at US hospitals" (Eisenberg et al., "Unconventional" 246). This blanket definition encompassed interventions ranging from self-administered practices such as meditation and prayer to fully institutionalized and accredited health systems such as massage therapy and chiropractic. Eisenberg and colleagues stunned the medical community by revealing that during the survey year

(1990), Americans' total number of visits to alternative health practitioners far outstripped those to conventional primary doctors (427 million visits and 388 million respectively). The Eisenberg survey signaled that the landscape of American medicine had shifted dramatically, seemingly overnight. This survey fueled a push for scientific studies of CAM that would ramp up over the decade that followed.

After Eisenberg's study, research efforts increased slowly at first, as the medical profession came to grips with the public's newfound interest in health practices that many perceived as more natural and holistic than mainstream medicine. The Office of Alternative Medicine, established by the National Institutes of Health in 1992, incubated some of the early research on CAM, although its starting annual budget of only $2 million limited its reach. By mid-decade, however, CAM had fully entered the medical profession's collective consciousness. In 1996, when editorial board members and staff of the *Journal of the American Medical Association* (*JAMA*) and its nine associated *Archives* specialty journals voted on the theme of their annual coordinated issues, they ranked alternative medicine sixty-eighth out of seventy-three possible themes. That same year, regular readers of *JAMA* ranked alternative medicine dramatically higher, at seventh among the same seventy-three topics, according to a concurrent survey of a stratified sample of readers led by the journal's then-editor George Lundberg (Lundberg, Paul, and Fritz). The following year, in 1997, the journals' editorial staff and board members likewise ranked CAM highly as a potential theme, at third out of eighty-six, and selected it as the topic for the following year's coordinated issues (Fontanarosa and Lundberg, "Call for Papers" 2111).

Published in November 1998, the coordinated CAM-themed issues of *JAMA* and the *Archives* represented the first significant step toward concerted, large-scale scientific scrutiny of once-fringe health practices such as acupuncture and herbal supplements and remedies. The theme issues' coordinating editors, Phil Fontanarosa and George Lundberg, described the CAM-themed journals as representing a historic moment for the medical profession. Although the journals, published at arm's-length by the American Medical Association (AMA), coordinate theme issues every year, the editors argued that the 1998 installment would be unique because it offered medical researchers and practitioners a "multidisciplinary forum" for sharing research on unconventional health practices in a space typically reserved for conventional biomedicine (Fontanarosa and Lundberg, "Call for Papers" 2111). Not all contributors to the journals favored such a multidisciplinary approach, however. Tom Delbanco, for instance, a professor at Harvard Medical School, equated research on CAM to the "scientific study of astrology," maintaining in a *JAMA* editorial that "we are in the midst of a fad that will pass" (1561). Delbanco, along with other commentators at the time, worried that biomedicine had succumbed to external pressures—pressures to which many had believed medicine immune.

But medicine was not immune: the AMA journals' 1998 concurrent theme issues on CAM were emblematic of the wider shift in medical culture that occurred over the final decade of the twentieth century, as CAM edged toward the mainstream. Large American university hospitals opened integrative medicine centers offering various alternative modalities and many medical schools tweaked their curricula to offer students rudimentary training in CAM principles and practices, to help them to advise patients who were interested in alternative medicine. Just months before the AMA journals published the CAM-themed issues, the National Institutes of Health transformed its tiny Office of Alternative Medicine into the full-fledged National Center for Complementary and Alternative Medicine. This new national research center dedicated its $50 million starting annual budget to fostering scientific scrutiny of CAM interventions and collaboration with CAM practitioners. At the turn of the twenty-first century, then, CAM appeared poised to enter the mainstream.

The potential impact on the medical profession of this wider cultural shift in health and health care was not lost on Fontanarosa and Lundberg, the theme issue editors. In their call for papers, they asserted that the journals would be taking a bold new step by briefly opening the closely monitored territory of mainstream scientific medicine to health practices normally beyond the scope of such journals. Prior to 1998, occasional articles on CAM practices such as acupuncture and chiropractic had long been published in mainstream medical journals. In *JAMA* alone, an article calling for clinical trials of acupuncture had been published some twenty-five years earlier, prompting several years of debate about the methodological and professional repercussions of such trials (Adler). However, as Fontanarosa and Lundberg recognized, what distinguished the *JAMA-Archives* coordinated theme issues from previous medical publications on CAM is their critical mass—their deliberate orchestration as an intensive, public meditation on CAM offered across a professional organization's network of texts.

The gravity of this rhetorical moment registered widely both within the medical community and beyond. It led, for example, to sustained debates in the medical literature about the theme issues' long-term implications for the profession as the lines between mainstream and alternative appeared to begin to blur. Media outlets such as *Newsweek* and *PBS Frontline* framed the research on CAM as historic, with the November 24, 2002, cover of *Newsweek* heralding the dawn of the "new science" of alternative medicine. Even the AMA journals commemorated the theme issues in 2000 by publishing the substantial volume *Alternative Medicine: An Objective Assessment*, a 600-page edited collection of articles from the 1998 journals (Fontanarosa, ed.). Recalling the theme issues' aftermath, Lundberg told me in an email in August 2014 that the journals had been so controversial within the medical community that, when he was fired very publicly by the AMA as *JAMA*'s editor in January 1999 after seventeen years in the position, many attributed his dismissal, in whole or in part, to his decision to publish the CAM theme issues two months earlier (Lundberg; see also Horton).[1]

In this book, I argue that the publication of the coordinated CAM-themed issues of *JAMA* and the *Archives* constitutes an important rhetorical moment in the production and maintenance of medical-professional boundaries. As CAM practices were subjected for the first time to concerted, large-scale scientific scrutiny, the rhetorical moment that unfolded in the *JAMA-Archives* was marked by a sense of disciplinary anxiety, with practitioners both within biomedicine and beyond struggling to identify their positions vis-à-vis this awkward union of different health models, which I will categorize loosely for now as *mainstream* and *alternative*.[2] In *JAMA* and the *Archives*, we do not see an effort to connect models of health and health care as much as a conflict over turf—a conflict between the dominant medical paradigm (mainstream medicine) and that ostensibly formed in opposition to it (alternative medicine). The theme issues' primary legacy for scholars interested in the rhetorical dimensions of biomedical boundaries therefore lies in the fact that the journals appear ultimately to have produced a reinvigorated status quo, wherein the borders separating what counts as mainstream medicine from what does not have not been erased, but instead have been bolstered significantly by scientific research.

Rhetoric at the Fringes of Medicine

In the chapters that follow, I examine the coordinated *JAMA-Archives* theme issues and related medical and public commentaries from the decade surrounding their publication in order to provide an account of how a dominant system of thought and practice responds to externally motivated challenges to its authority. How, for instance, do members of the medical community respond discursively to pressure (even internal pressure) to integrate complementary and alternative practices into their own system of thought? And does that pressure, in turn, influence how biomedicine itself functions? For example, historian of medicine James Whorton cites the "biomedical reductionism" of conventional medicine (i.e., the reduction of persons to diseased bodies) as a major factor in the movement of patients toward CAM. Does that movement, in turn, motivate doctors to transform their own practice to accommodate patients that prefer care that is more attentive to their experiences of illness?

The conceptual, ethical, professional, and practical problems that arise in the scientific testing of CAM are problems of commensurability—the commensurability of theories, procedures, and evidence. Traditional Chinese medicine (TCM), for example, is founded on the principle of energy flow through channels, or meridians, that do not correspond to any physiological structure known to Western physicians. Given that biomedicine and TCM are premised on radically different models of bodies, illness, and health, biomedical researchers are faced with a fundamental problem regarding how they ought to proceed with scientific studies of TCM. To study TCM as a standardized treatment in double-blind, placebo-controlled trials would violate the principles that govern TCM—holistic, patient-specific care that unites physical, psychological, and spiritual elements of healing. But the methodological features of blinding, controlling, and standardizing are exactly what make scientific research scientific, and to alter those features to fit within the TCM framework would jeopardize the knowledge that such trials produce. It could also jeopardize the careers of the scientists conducting them.

To open up problems such as these to inquiry, I situate the *JAMA-Archives* theme issues in the context of rhetoric, the art and study of persuasion as it is enacted through processes both conscious and unconscious. Rhetorical analysis illuminates how we are induced, through symbolic and discursive means, toward certain beliefs and actions and away from others. Rhetoric scholars focus their attention on human communication and the webbed relations among knowledge, belief, language, argument, speakers, and audiences. Because rhetorical theory shows us how language shapes both our world and our understanding of it, rhetoric can take us a long way toward making sense of how biomedicine interacts with competing, and sometimes conflicting, approaches to health and health care.

From a rhetorical perspective, what is most important about the CAM-themed issues of *JAMA* and the *Archives* is not that their effects on the medical profession were lasting, although as I suggest in the conclusion, the journals do appear to have helped in the "mainstreaming" of CAM (Ruggie). Rather, for the purposes of this book, what is most important about the journals is the self-conscious nature of their production. Even though the contributors held varied positions on CAM research (some in favor, some not), the authors collectively saw the publication of the theme issues as a significant opportunity for their profession's self-fashioning.

In the preface to the edited volume of essays based on the theme issues, published in 2000, for instance, the AMA's then-president Thomas Reardon noted the significance of the *JAMA-Archives'* efforts for medicine as a whole: "This [collection] is a milestone. The authors and editors delineate where the science begins and ends as of today, outlining where further study is needed" (v). Reardon makes it no secret that the *JAMA-Archives'* efforts to delineate a biomedical science of CAM were explicitly rhetorical, centered on persuasion: they were aimed at deliberation about what sort of enterprise medicine is and ought to be.[3] If current evidence suggesting a sharp drop in Americans' expenditure and use of CAM is any indication, those deliberative efforts appear, a decade and a half later, not to have been in vain.[4]

One of this book's broader claims is that the study of rhetoric at the fringes of medicine is illuminating for both medicine and rhetoric. Rhetoric helps us to investigate fringe patients, fringe illnesses, fringe practitioners, and fringe health models—to study the means through which they fail, somehow, to fit within the accepted boundaries of mainstream scientific medicine. Such medical fringes, in turn, offer to rhetorical theory productive ways of tracking what sociologist Thomas Gieryn calls the "boundary work" of science: they focus attention on the shifting border between what is deemed legitimate within science and what is not. The central premise of this book is that the means through which medical researchers solve the professional and epistemological problems they face in their research on CAM are boundary-focused and largely rhetorical, centered on persuasion.

I extend earlier studies of biomedicine's fraught engagement with complementary and alternative medicine by beginning my analysis from the position that the shifting divisions between modes of health care are the product not only of historical or social processes, such as professional regulation or market competition, but of processes that are inherently rhetorical: the preservation or destruction of the categories of mainstream and alternative must themselves be effected through persuasive means. The solutions that researchers adopt in their studies of unconventional health practices persuade us in various directions—they persuade us about biomedicine's scope and limits; about the status and legitimacy of specific CAM practices; about what counts as a contribution to knowledge; and about how we understand our own illness and health. This process of coping with external challenges, I maintain, constitutes a particularly intense episode of "edging and filling" of scientific boundaries, in Gieryn's terms, and is a useful place to isolate and describe some of the rhetorical constituents of boundary work within medicine.

Mapping Biomedical Boundaries

Contemporary Western medicine is shaped predominantly by the biomedical model, which medical anthropologist Howard Stein notes has its roots in the "basic sciences" of anatomy, biochemistry, microbiology, pathology, and physiology (xiv). As a descriptive term, *biomedicine* does not refer to a fully fixed set of medical values or practices but, as Stein explains, certain overarching tenets do characterize the ways in which medicine is conceptualized and taught in the United States, Canada, and elsewhere. These tenets include the principles that medicine is, and ought to be, predicated on "rational, scientific, dispassionate, objective, professional judgment"; that the causes of disease are rooted in organic pathology, typically at the cellular level; and that disease is "optimally" treated by interventions resulting in a cure (xiv).

The shape of medical research, teaching, and practice are determined largely by the biomedical disciplines (e.g., cardiology, dermatology, and endocrinology) that are structured around organ systems. These defining qualities of biomedicine place it squarely within the province of science, although numerous critics have demonstrated how this essentially mechanistic approach occludes medicine's humanistic core (see, e.g., Murray; Peabody). While CAM practices are not themselves biomedical, the shape and scope they hold in Western culture is nevertheless determined significantly by how they are configured in relation to biomedicine and, in turn, to science.

Some fifty years ago, philosophers of science Thomas Kuhn and Paul Feyerabend observed, separately, that definitions of what science is depend entirely on context—historical, philosophical, epistemological, professional. In rhetorical terms, they depend on the sophistic notion of *kairos*, the elements of time, place, and circumstance. More recently, Gieryn has similarly described science in cartographic terms, as a bounded cultural space that is neither permanent nor rigidly defined but that is nevertheless carefully protected and patrolled. He argues that "The epistemic authority of science is . . . , through repeated and endless edging and filling of its boundaries, sustained over lots of local situations and episodic moments, but 'science' never takes on exactly the same shape or contents from contest to contest" (*Cultural Boundaries* 14). The routine maintenance of science's boundaries makes up much of what Kuhn calls normal science, including the day-to-day accumulation of facts and figures in labs, observatories, and the field. All of the data that scientists produce are interpreted, sorted, and sifted; results are tabulated and deemed significant or not, and conclusions are devised. All of these are, *inter alia*, rhetorical processes.[5]

Central to Kuhn's and Feyerabend's theoretical treatises on scientific knowledge is the notion of incommensurability, the lack of a common measure or standard by which to judge competing accounts of nature. Kuhn's classic example of incommensurability is the lack of a common standard between the Ptolemaic universe and the Copernican: as long as one sees the universe as centered on Earth, a sun-centered world can never make sense. Biomedical research on CAM faces similar problems of commensurability because the theoretical foundations of many alternative practices are incompatible with biomedicine's pathophysiological core. Practices such as Ayurveda, chiropractic, and traditional Chinese medicine, for example, center on principles of energy flow and balance, but they find no such corollary in biomedicine. These principles are therefore incommensurable with the clinical trial framework. The notion of incommensurability articulates a framework that, for our present purposes, helps us understand the concrete obstacles in CAM research that affect our ability to test, through scientific methods, health practices not based on the scientific model.

Since Kuhn and Feyerabend, the notion of incommensurability has captured the attention of historians and philosophers of science, but, while it is a partly rhetorical problem, rhetoricians have taken it up only recently. Adopting I. A. Richards's definition of rhetoric as the "study of misunderstanding and its remedies" as a rallying cry, Randy Allen Harris assembled in 2005 some of the most important scholars in rhetoric of science to spin out the implications of incommensurability for rhetoric, and vice versa. Defining incommensurability as "a phenomenon of misaligned meanings [in context]" (Introduction, *Rhetoric* 59), Harris argues that although incommensurability should be disabling for science, it is not; his contributors investigate why this is so.

Several chapters in Harris's collection provide insight relevant to the study of the rhetoric of medical "fringes" because they trace incommensurability in science along synchronic, not diachronic, axes, examining conflict among contemporaneous paradigms rather than across successive ones. Carolyn Miller's chapter on the convergence of physical and biological sciences finds something like incommensurability ("Novelty and Heresy"), while Charles Bazerman and René Agustín De los Santos's chapter on toxicology and ecotoxicology does not. Leah Ceccarelli maps how the very notion of incommensurability can become entrenched as a model of scientific argument, wherein rhetors envision debate about scientific controversy as an agonistic struggle, a "zero-sum game" ("Science and Civil Debate" 274). While their conclusions differ, these authors usefully track potential conceptual and communicative problems in boundary-crossing research, and the possibilities for their resolution.

Other rhetorical studies of science by Leah Ceccarelli (*Shaping Science*), Greg Myers (*Writing Biology*), Charles Alan Taylor, and Greg Wilson and Carl Herndl share an interest in tracking boundary work—how different scientific specialties interface with one another. Taylor writes most directly on the demarcation of science from nonscience, a matter that he describes as thoroughly rhetorical: "demarcations of science are accomplished routinely in everyday social and scientific practice. . . . [S]uch demarcations proceed not from ontological foundations but from symbolic inducements. They are, then, rhetorical accomplishments" (15). Taylor surveys scholarship from history, philosophy, and sociology of science with the aim of developing a uniquely rhetorical account of demarcation. His two case studies on creation science and cold fusion illustrate that the demarcation of what counts as science is largely a "discursive accomplishment" emerging out of scientists' everyday practices (222).

Some researchers have investigated rhetorical boundary work specifically in biomedicine. Debra Journet's early study from 1993, for example, analyzed a prominent physician's attempts to manage the conflicting interests and expectations of his two key audiences—neurologists and psychoanalysts—for his theory of psychosomatic medicine. More recently, researchers have investigated the discursive boundaries of medicine as it intersects with both allied disciplines, such as science and business (Popham), and allied civic agencies, such as child protection services, police, and the courts (Spafford et al.). These studies advance our understanding of rhetorical boundary work within medicine but they examine tensions among those who are all, in an important sense, medical insiders. The texts analyzed in each article are situated firmly within the systems of knowledge and practice of mainstream Western (bio-) medicine. Further, they are united in the goal of fostering connections between disparate ways of thinking and acting.

Certain scholars have examined rhetorical boundary work closer to the edges of biomedicine, particularly as it concerns health practitioners and patients who do not fit easily within mainstream models of health care. Mary Lay Schuster and Philippa Spoel, for example, have separately traced the evolution of the once-fringe practice of midwifery in the US and Canada respectively, examining the strategies that midwives have adopted in their quest to gain autonomy as members of a health care profession.[6] Similarly, Judy Segal (*Health*, "Illness") has studied the rhetorical life of patients with nonspecific symptoms and symptoms without immediately recognizable biological causes (e.g., achiness, fatigue), who struggle to fit within biomedical conceptions of disease. These studies add to our understanding of how medical outsiders gain access to the mainstream system (or not).

Schuster's and Spoel's research on midwifery focuses on reproduction, itself an important area of study in the rhetoric of medical boundary work, since medicine is conventionally understood as the treatment of illness, a category into which childbearing does not fit neatly. However, their focus on midwifery leaves open the question of how *primary* CAM modalities, such as TCM and chiropractic, which advocate comprehensive systems of care, come into contact with biomedicine. What sorts of "misaligned meanings," in Harris's formulation, arise at such points of contact? How, for instance, do essentially competing approaches to health, based on apparently incommensurable understandings of bodies, illness, and health, find any common ground? And while Schuster, Segal, and Spoel all provide accounts of how fringe patients/illnesses/practices enter into those encounters with biomedicine, there is still the question of how mainstream medicine, as the dominant system of knowledge and practice in North American health care, responds to challenges to its borders—and, by extension, to challenges to its social and epistemic authority.

This book addresses such questions and extends our knowledge of rhetorical boundary work by isolating five key dimensions of persuasion in the production and maintenance of biomedicine's boundaries as they operate within the *JAMA-Archives* theme issues and their surrounding medical and public discourse. I demonstrate that biomedicine is bounded by (1) how the notion of evidence defines and circumscribes the limits of acceptable knowledge; (2) how medical researchers and practitioners define and categorize the practices that comprise CAM; (3) how researchers design and interpret clinical studies; (4) how those studies configure practitioner-patient interaction; and (5) how the evidence produced by those studies is reported to the public. Each of these five dimensions of biomedical boundary work comprises a chapter of this book, which together fill in the picture of how biomedicine comes to and maintains ascendancy over other health practices and practitioners.

Central to each of these five dimensions of boundary work is the notion of evidence and how that notion functions rhetorically in different contexts for different purposes. As I explain in chapter 1, biomedical debates about the legitimacy of CAM practices such as acupuncture and chiropractic generally hinge on whether or not there is sufficient evidence of their safety and efficacy. But that evidence does not emerge, free of conflict or context, directly out of research settings. Instead, research data are transformed as they move from labs and clinics out into the wider world, qualifying as "evidence" only once validated in peer-reviewed journals under the imprimatur of established medical organizations and publishers. On the question of evidence in biomedical boundaries, then, journals such as *JAMA* and the *Archives* are the sites where that evidence originates and, thus, they constitute the primary point of inquiry for understanding how the medical profession negotiates its limits vis-à-vis complementary and alternative medicine.

To plumb the five dimensions of boundary work outlined above as they operate in the *JAMA-Archives* theme issues, I have organized this book around a key question that forms the throughline for the chapters that follow: *How does the notion of evidence determine the boundaries of biomedicine, from expert to public contexts?* In focusing on evidence in debates about CAM, I am less concerned with how doctors *know* whether or not CAM is safe and effective than with how they *demonstrate*, both to themselves and to others, how they know—and in turn, how those demonstrations of knowledge, in the form of "evidence," influence biomedicine's limits. What I show is that the concept of evidence is fraught and variable, and can be deployed differently in different contexts to achieve particular ends, even when those deploying it intend only to produce useful, objective knowledge about the world. In debates about complementary and alternative medicine, recourse to the notion of evidence determines not only what counts as safe and effective medicine: it also, simultaneously, determines what belongs within or beyond the boundaries of biomedicine.

Analyzing a Rhetorical Moment

My analysis of the rhetorical moment captured in the 1998 CAM-themed issues of *JAMA* and the *Archives* centers on the theme issues themselves, which comprise approximately eighty articles, across all ten of the journals published by the American Medical Association (table 1). The journals offer varying degrees of coverage of the CAM theme: *JAMA* is entirely devoted to the theme and all of the major articles in *Archives of Internal Medicine* are on CAM. *Archives of Dermatology* and *Archives of Family Medicine* each dedicate about half of their pages to the shared theme. *Archives of Neurology* and *Archives of Pediatrics and Adolescent Medicine* feature several articles on CAM intermixed with articles on conventional topics, whereas *Archives of Surgery* lists its CAM articles separately under the heading "Special Articles." Other journals offer little, if any, coverage on the shared theme: *Archives of General Psychiatry* offers only two articles on CAM, while *Archives of Otolaryngology—Head and Neck Surgery* offers one, and *Archives of Ophthalmology*, none.

The articles within the journals take a variety of forms, including preliminary research reports, original reports of randomized controlled trials (RCTs), systematic reviews (metastudies of RCTs), review articles, editorials and commentaries, letters, news briefs, and essays on medical ethics, pol-

TABLE 1. List of the AMA-published journals and theme issues

Journal	Theme issue
Journal of the American Medical Association	November 11, 1998 (vol. 208, no. 18)
Archives of Dermatology	November 1998 (vol. 134, no. 11)
Archives of Family Medicine	November/December 1998 (vol. 7, no. 6)
Archives of General Psychiatry	November 1998 (vol. 55, no. 11)
Archives of Internal Medicine	November 9, 1998 (vol. 158, no. 20)
Archives of Neurology	November 1998 (vol. 55, no. 11)
Archives of Ophthalmology	November 1998 (vol. 116, no. 11)
Archives of Otolaryngology—Head & Neck Surgery	November 1998 (vol. 124, no. 11)
Archives of Pediatrics & Adolescent Medicine	November 1998 (vol. 152, no. 11)
Archives of Surgery	November 1998 (vol. 133, no. 11)

icy, and practice. All of the articles are organized and published within the journals' regular sections and categories (e.g., "News and Views," "Original Contributions," "A Piece of My Mind"), which vary by publication. These categorizations and the distribution of CAM-related articles under them are visible in the table of contents from the *JAMA* theme issue, illustrated in figure 1.

I analyze the theme issues through methods drawn primarily from rhetorical theory and criticism. The term *rhetoric* is often understood to refer to empty or deceptive speech—"mere" rhetoric, rather than language conveying truth or action. While this description certainly applies to some instances of persuasive language use, rhetoric is more broadly an ancient body of theory and practice advanced by figures such as Plato, Aristotle, Cicero, and others, who held the art of persuasive discourse as central to public life. Since the classical period, rhetoric has expanded beyond the language of the agora into a full-bodied field of inquiry on the production and reception of discourse, written and spoken, verbal and visual. In its contemporary form as a discipline at the nexus of the humanities and social sciences, *rhetoric* is both a critical-hermeneutic and an empirical practice that centers on persuasion, on all of the ways in which we act on each other (and ourselves) by influence, through methods both conscious and unconscious, through various communicative means. In studying how texts are put together to achieve their effects, rhetoricians often appear to imply premeditated calculation on the author's part. But this is an appearance, only: as Leah Ceccarelli points out, "Just as an organism might adopt a successful evolutionary strategy without being consciously aware of it, so too might an author adopt a successful rhetorical strategy without being consciously aware of it" (*Shaping Science* 5).

November 11, 1998, Vol 280, No. 18 Pages 1549-1640

To promote the science and art of medicine and the betterment of the public health.

(Table of Contents continued on next page.)

FIGURE 1. Table of contents, *Journal of the American Medical Association* 280.18 (1998): 1549–50.

Within the larger theoretical framework of rhetoric, I situate my analysis of the *JAMA-Archives* theme issues in rhetoric of health and medicine, a vibrant and growing but diverse subfield in rhetorical studies that developed, partially, out of rhetoric of science. The subfield is recently coming into its own, with an increasing presence in graduate programs and academic journals and conferences, as well as in recent field-mapping monographs and collections (e.g., Segal, *Health*; Heifferon and Brown, eds.; Leach and Dysart-Gale, eds.) and specialized monographs on rhetorics of breastfeeding (Koerber), depression (Emmons), pain (Graham), pregnancy (Seigel), psychiatric case histories (Berkenkotter, *Patient Tales*), and research misconduct (Keränen). Research in this subfield overlaps with diverse other fields, including other areas of language study such as composition studies, health communication, linguistic-pragmatics, and professional and technical communication.

Often, distinctions among these language-based approaches can be difficult to make, as Segal's survey of the variety of scholarship in rhetoric of health and medicine illustrates ("Rhetoric of Health and Medicine").[7] Scholarship in rhetoric of health and medicine also borrows from, contributes to, and overlaps with other disciplines such as anthropology, history, philosophy, and sociology, and interdisciplinary research areas such as bioethics, health/medical humanities, medicine studies, and science studies.

In my analysis of the *JAMA-Archives* theme issues in the chapters that follow, I take what Blake Scott calls "a rhetorical-cultural approach" ("Extending," *Risky*). Such an approach incorporates methods from both rhetoric and cultural studies, although, as Marika Seigel notes, "This perspective does not mean forgoing rhetorical analysis, but it does mean reading texts less as rhetorical productions of intentional agents, or authors. Instead, rhetorical-cultural analysis emphasizes a text's conditions of possibility and its possible rhetorical and material effects" (22).[8] Following this approach, in my research for this book, I read all of the articles within the *JAMA-Archives* theme issues, as well as related discursive artifacts on the theme issues such as their calls for papers, earlier scholarly articles that were prominently cited within them, letters to the editor, and all later articles within the scholarly literature, across disciplines, that reflected on their significance within and for the medical profession. I also read general commentaries about CAM published in other medical journals and popular news media coverage of the research reported in *JAMA* and the *Archives*. Alongside these articles, I examined relevant scholarship in fields such as history, philosophy, sociology, and medicine to attain a broader understanding of biomedicine's entanglements with complementary and alternative medicine. Much of my reading of this scholarship centered on medicine as a field of research and practice, as a profession, and as a culture. Patient beliefs, experience, and behavior figured prominently in my reading as well.

The key aims of rhetorical-cultural analysis of science, in Scott's view, are "accounting for science's broader conditions of possibility, mapping the shifting intertext of science in action, evaluating science according to its effects, and targeting opportunities to intervene in harmful effects" (*Risky* 21). Following on these aims, the goal of my analysis of the CAM-themed issues of *JAMA* and the *Archives* was not principally to better understand the theme issues themselves but to understand both the context out of which they emerged and their subsequent effects on the communities of knowledge and practice associated with them. In keeping with Scott's approach, I strive in this book to "intervene in harmful effects" relevant to biomedical boundary work, but I do so not through prescription but through description: this book opens up for inquiry the means through which biomedical boundaries are effected through persuasion and are themselves persuasive; I do not, in my analysis, adjudicate on whether or how those boundaries ought to be.

In terms of my analytic method, the chapter descriptions below include the specific rhetorical constructs I employ, such as constitutive rhetoric, genre theory, and rhetorical *topoi*, or topics. I augmented these constructs with other research methods to more effectively map "the shifting intertext of science" vis-à-vis biomedical boundary work and to corroborate my textual analysis of the *JAMA-Archives* theme issues. Following Ceccarelli (*Shaping Science*), I tested my hypotheses about the texts' rhetorical effects, where possible, by examining published responses to those texts in subsequent discursive activities such as follow-up articles in *JAMA*, the *Archives*, and other scholarly and popular publications. I also draw on others' empirical research throughout the book, which I consulted in a comparative process to ground my own analysis, as when I use observational research on practitioner-patient interaction in traditional Chinese medicine and chiropractic to corroborate my investigation of how such interaction is configured in randomized controlled trials of those practices.

I also conducted discourse-based interviews with five health professionals from three areas of expertise: two medical researchers, two practitioners of traditional Chinese medicine (TCM), and one physician-clinician. The two medical researchers, both experts in trial design, worked at a hospital-based, multidisciplinary center for clinical epidemiology, which, in addition to its own research mandate, offered a consulting service on trial design and evidence interpretation. The TCM practitioners also spanned the career spectrum, and both maintained active clinical practices. The physician-clinician was a midcareer doctor maintaining a busy family practice specializing in obstetrical care. These interviews form the substantive basis of my analysis of two randomized controlled trials of acupuncture published in the *JAMA* theme issue, which I discuss in chapter 2, and they bolster my discussion elsewhere in the book, particularly in chapter 3.[9]

The purpose of the interviews was to learn how readers with different professional orientations would respond to the studies' methods and designs. Although the sample size is too small to draw generalizations about attitudes held by populations of such readers, the responses elicited do offer insight into the different kinds of concerns that individual readers bring to boundary-crossing scientific texts. The interviews followed Odell, Goswami, and Herrington's discourse-based interview method, in which participants read aloud from a specific text and report, in real time, on their processes of writing or reading, depending on the focus of the research. The interviews unfolded in two stages for each article without a predefined set of questions. For the first stage of each article, participants read aloud from one excerpt from the methods section and one from the results section, and were asked to interrupt their reading at any time to comment if something struck them as noteworthy. Any such commentary was further explored through general prompts such as "Would most people in your field agree with/say that?" as well as prompts particular to each reader's area of expertise.[10] The second stage for each article focused on the article as a whole, prompted with the question, "Are there any other aspects of the articles that you would like to comment on?" Each interview lasted about an hour and was concluded when the participant had no further comments or concerns. The participants were not aware of the articles' inclusion in the *JAMA-Archives* theme issues on CAM until they were debriefed at the end of the interviews. Audiorecordings of these interviews were transcribed verbatim and analyzed both to guide my own analysis and to provide data regarding how different readers interpreted the studies' design and results differently.

The diverse analytic methods I employ in this book enable me to examine a discrete discursive moment from multiple perspectives, at multiple levels of analysis. As a work of rhetorical criticism, this book takes an unusual approach to its material because, rather than shifting its object of analysis with each chapter while employing the same or similar methods throughout the text, the book applies *different* methods to the *same* object—or set of objects. This approach yields new insight for our understanding of medical discourse because the approach operates very much in the manner of the randomized controlled trial (RCT) in medical research: whereas RCTs control all aspects of an experimental study except the variable under investigation (usually a pharmaceutical), which is then manipulated under various conditions to examine the variable's effects, each chapter of this book investigates the same rhetorical moment (the variable under study) through a different perspective to reveal a different dimension of boundary work. I describe below these different perspectives and the effects of the *JAMA-Archives* theme issues under each. Such an approach produces a more complete understanding than has been afforded by previous scholarship on the rhetorical means through which medical researchers and practitioners maintain the bounds of their profession.

Preview of Chapters

The progress and shape of this book can be described in rhetorician Kenneth Burke's metaphor of photographic filters. Describing his theory of "terministic screens," Burke explains:

> I have particularly in mind some photographs I once saw. They were *different* photographs of the *same* objects, the difference being that they were made with different color filters. Here something so "factual" as a photograph revealed notable distinctions in texture, and even in form, depending on which color filter was used for the documentary description of the event being recorded. (*Language* 45; original emphasis)

I approach the coordinated CAM-themed issues of *JAMA* and the *Archives* as a set of snapshots of the medical profession's discursive activity at a single historical moment, as it negotiated what counts as safe and effective health care and what does not. In the first chapter, I set up the background and main arguments that I advance in this book, while each of the remaining chapters examine biomedical boundary work in the *JAMA-Archives* theme issues through different "filters": historical-professional, epistemological, clinical, and public. Together, the chapters move from professional (i.e., internal) concerns to public (external) concerns about biomedical research on CAM. The first three chapters examine what Bruno Latour has called the "upstream" activities of scientists, while the remaining two chapters heed Gieryn's call for studies of science as it moves "downstream" into the public realm, where the borders of biomedicine are all the more apparent in their juxtaposition with everyday human life. In the manner of Burke's photographic filters, each chapter reveals different elements of medicine—and of rhetoric.

As noted earlier, this book is organized around a central question: *How does the notion of evidence determine the boundaries of biomedicine, from expert to public contexts?* In chapter 1, I lay the groundwork for answering this question, first by explaining what I mean by "evidence" and by "boundaries," and then by illustrating how both terms accrue rhetorical significance within biomedicine. I key the CAM-themed issues of *JAMA* and the *Archives* to the emergence of evidence-based medicine as a qualitatively new model of medical practice, in which primarily quantitative data from clinical trials abstract medical decision-making from the physicians and researchers who engage in it. I show in this chapter how recourse to "the evidence" in debates about complementary and alternative health interventions can operate as a strategy of exclusion, wherein arguments about whether or not a given health practice is safe and effective are embedded within the medical-disciplinary matrices out of which they emerge.

Chapter 2 examines how the contributors to the CAM-themed issues of *JAMA* and the *Archives* situate their texts, on subjects not typically under the purview of such journals, in relation to the historical-professional dynamics that have shaped biomedicine. I examine the coordinated theme issues as textual artifacts within the context of professional discourse to show how they reframe both biomedicine and CAM in terms that preserve biomedicine's historical coherence as a firmly defined discipline while simultaneously stretching its limits to reach practices formerly beyond its scope. This process serves inherently epideictic functions, reinforcing conventional community values and the perceived borders separating health practices, even while some community members ostensibly seek to eradicate those borders.

Chapter 3 focuses on method—ways of doing or procedures for acting—as the key rhetorical *topos*, or topic, that furnishes lines of argument that researchers adopt to align CAM practices with scientific borders. At the core of these journals is an epistemological debate about how research on CAM ought to be conducted, interpreted, and incorporated into practice because biomedicine's "gold standard" methodology, the randomized controlled trial (RCT), does not easily accommodate interventions such as acupuncture. I examine how CAM practices fit awkwardly within the RCT format and, turning to studies of the rhetoric of experimental articles in both science and medicine, I investigate how the experimental genre is mobilized in the specific case of biomedical CAM research. I then isolate the concept of *efficacy*—whether or not a health intervention "works"—as a central organizing principle of biomedical research on CAM. I show that efficacy can be invoked strategically to draw particular epistemic and professional boundary lines. As this chapter argues, the problem of method in biomedical CAM research is largely a problem of persuasion: the ways that researchers design their studies and report their findings determine which health interventions belong in biomedicine and which do not.

Central to the question of methodology in CAM research is the practitioner-patient relationship, the most unambiguously rhetorical element of clinical medicine. Increased interaction between practitioners and patients in any medical model may have unintended—and unquantifiable—therapeutic effects. Chapter 4 examines how the *JAMA-Archives* theme issues and related textual artifacts configure practitioner-patient interaction, particularly in relation to prevalent models of medical practice. I argue that the these texts posit practitioner-patient interaction as a potential contaminant in trials of acupuncture and chiropractic, wherein attempts to control for placebo effects are, in many cases, attempts to control for interaction effects. I suggest that probing these interaction effects can facilitate new understandings of how practitioner-patient encounters can influence health outcomes. Finally, I examine the idea of patient autonomy, closely linked to interaction and central to discourses about CAM in both the texts under study and the medical literature more generally. I argue that the actual extent of autonomy afforded to patients in medical settings, alternative or not, is often illusory, framed within generic and rhetorical processes that necessarily tilt the course of decision-making in particular, and predictably biomedical, directions.

The final chapter, chapter 5, shifts further downstream into the public realm, to examine popular reporting on biomedical research on CAM, particularly a special report in *Newsweek* magazine on the "new science of alternative medicine." I articulate a rhetoric of popular medicine vis-à-vis theoretical models of popular science developed in rhetoric, discourse studies, and social studies of science to argue that health reporting is both typical of and exceptional in science reporting: it is typical because medicine's research values, generic forms, and institutional structures are closely aligned with those of science, yet it is exceptional because members of the public are significantly more invested as a rhetorical audience of medical reporting, due both to their own bodily experience and expertise and to their need for health information. I further suggest that CAM research demonstrates the bidirectional nature of science reporting, in contrast to the unidirectional model proposed by earlier theorists, because the major push for CAM research was motivated, in the first instance, by overwhelming public interest in and use of CAM therapies. In the texts from *Newsweek* that I study in this chapter, the products of that research are returned, transformed by science into statistical outcomes, to the public that motivated it.

This book moves in an arc that begins with internal boundary-defining documents in medicine—in this case, the letters, editorials, and research reports published in, and in response to, *JAMA* and the *Archives*—and ends with how such boundary work ultimately informs rhetorical interaction among health professions, professionals, and the public, although, as I suggest in chapter 5, this process is at least partly bidirectional. The study of the discursive boundaries between mainstream and alternative medicine explores, simultaneously, a host of related boundaries, all of which can be illuminated by rhetorical study. These illuminated discursive boundaries return something to rhetoric as a whole: they offer a rhetorical account of how science and medicine, protectors of what Randy Allen Harris calls "the most robust knowledge of our culture" (Introduction, *Landmark Essays* xxix), shape—and are shaped by—the particularized experience of everyday human life.

Evidence, Rhetoric, and Disciplinary Boundaries

In their editorial accompanying the 1998 theme issue of the *Journal of the American Medical Association* (*JAMA*), editors Phil Fontanarosa and George Lundberg stake their claim in the debate over complementary and alternative medicine (CAM). The position they express in that editorial encapsulates what I argue in this book is a virtually invisible process, wherein the medical profession's explicit and self-conscious efforts to define its borders appear seamless, couched within an evidence-based terminology that defines CAM only in terms of what it is not:

> There is no alternative medicine. There is only scientifically proven, evidence-based medicine supported by solid data or unproven medicine, for which scientific evidence is lacking. Whether a therapeutic practice is "Eastern" or "Western,' is unconventional or mainstream, or involves mind-body techniques or molecular genetics is largely irrelevant except for historical purposes and cultural interest. We recognize that there are vastly different types of practitioners and proponents of the various forms of alternative medicine and conventional medicine, and that there are vast differences in the skills, capabilities, and beliefs of individuals within them and the nature of their actual practices. Moreover, the economic and political forces in these fields are large and increasingly complex and have the capability for being highly contentious. Nonetheless, as believers in science and evidence, we must focus on fundamental issues—namely, the patient, the target disease or condition, the proposed or practiced treatment, and the need for convincing data on safety and therapeutic efficacy. (Fontanarosa and Lundberg, "Alternative Medicine" 1618)

From the perspective of biomedical boundary work, there is much one could say about this editorial statement, which figures CAM simply as medicine that has not (or not yet) been proven by science to be effective and safe.

For one, this statement creates sharp lines of community membership. The final sentence, headed by the group-defining modifier "as believers in science and evidence," implies that those excluded from the "we" category of the main clause ("*we* must focus on fundamental issues . . .") do not value patients, targeting diseases, or the safety and efficacy of their treatments. Framed in terms of audience design, the linguistic theory of how speakers assign various roles to hearers, we might then read that sentence as saying something like: "*we*, those of us that read and publish in *JAMA*, believe these things, while other people, *out there*, do not necessarily." Framed in similar but more conventionally rhetorical terms, we could say that this final sentence fosters identification among its readers as "believers" in science and evidence, reinforcing their division from those who do not share such beliefs, such as those who value alternative medicine *as* an alternative to mainstream medicine.[1] It is worth noting, too, that science is invoked in this passage as a unitary concept, a heterogeneous set of epistemological and material research practices, when we might better consider it, in Gieryn's sense, as a culturally demarcated space.

The passage above also casually neutralizes a contentious subject by substituting a whole discourse—here captured in the expansive binaries of East versus West, unconventional versus mainstream, and mind-body versus molecular—with a new, single binary: proven versus unproven. In adopting this binary, the editors gloss over the role that extrascientific factors play in shaping biomedical boundaries, including conceptions of "Eastern" and "Western," different philosophies of health and illness, patient behaviors and preferences, and economic, political, regulatory, and institutional forces. Such a neutralizing effect is a common feature of language in both medical and scientific writing (Segal, "Strategies"; Martha Solomon). However, for an editorial introducing a potentially controversial topic such as CAM within a set of leading medical journals, the editors' approach is incongruous: one might more readily have expected a defensive tone or proleptic approach, with the editors anticipating and heading off readers' potential objections to the appearance of CAM in a mainstream scientific venue. The incongruity between the editors' matter-of-fact language and their potentially controversial topic calls our attention to the conditions in medicine that make it possible to introduce a collection of provocative editorials and methodologically challenging studies with such a clear-cut approach. Fontanarosa and Lundberg make the issue of testing alternative medicine sound so simple, as though the researchers' work were straightforward—to "prove" which treatments work and which do not, and then we will be able to do away with the alternative medicine debate once and for all.

This refrain, that we simply need more and better evidence on the safety and efficacy of alternative health interventions, is repeated frequently not only in *JAMA* and the *Archives* but also in the wider medical literature on CAM. Just two months prior to the publication of the 1998 theme issues, for example, Marcia Angell, then the executive editor of the preeminent *New England Journal of Medicine*, and her then-editor-in-chief, Jerome Kassirer, similarly declared that evidence, and only evidence, would end debates about CAM:

> There is only medicine that has been adequately tested and medicine that has not, medicine that works and medicine that may or may not work. Once a treatment has been tested rigorously, it no longer matters whether it was considered alternative at the outset. If it is found to be reasonably safe and effective, it will be accepted. But assertions, speculation, and testimonials do not substitute for evidence. Alternative treatments should be subjected to scientific testing no less rigorous than that required for conventional treatments. (841)

Angell and Kassirer's claim here, that rigorous scientific testing will give us the evidence we need to assess alternative health interventions, is virtually identical to that advanced by Fontanarosa and Lundberg in their *JAMA* editorial. Both of these examples illustrate that, in cases where medicine's boundaries are up for negotiation, the notion of evidence and the science that produces it carry an argumentative weight that can ultimately reshape the landscape of biomedicine by determining which health practices are deemed legitimate and which are not.

In this chapter, I establish and contextualize my core argument in this book that biomedicine is bounded, in the first instance, by how the notion of evidence defines and circumscribes the limits of acceptable knowledge. I develop this argument over the remaining chapters by tracking how the concept of evidence moves from the upstream realm of medical research down into the realms of medical practice and public discourse. Over the sections of this chapter, I explain the rising prominence in biomedicine of a particular understanding of evidence as primarily quantitative, derived not from clinical intuition or experience but from experimental studies that measure and compare interventions through scientific processes. The apparent objectivity of evidence produced through randomized controlled trials is one of the primary means through which the *JAMA-Archives* theme issues on CAM invisibly shift, and then seek to fix, the boundaries between what counts as proper medical science and what does not.

Recounting several earlier episodes of biomedical boundary work in the

United States, I show how recourse to "the evidence" in debates about the safety and efficacy of various CAM interventions can function as a strategy of exclusion, serving purposes that can, at times, be as much social and professional (and economic) as they are medical. These historical episodes do not merely provide background to the chapters that follow, however. Rather, they illustrate how claims regarding science's power to adjudicate on alternative medicine have evolved in such a way that the notion of evidence itself has become a moving target: there is always more and better evidence that could be obtained on a given health intervention. For many alternative health practices and practitioners, then, the threshold of sufficient evidence may be always just out of reach.

While the current weight of evidence in arguments about complementary and alternative health emerges out of a recent and qualitatively new understanding of what counts as data in medical research, that understanding is rooted in an evolutionary process that began with the rise of the medical profession itself. For all else that it is, the history of medicine is also a history of boundary work, a narrative of healthcare providers' efforts, both conscious and unconscious, to maintain and expand their territory within the professional ecosystem (Baer; R. Porter; Saks; Starr). Over the years, that boundary work has become less visible, naturalized with rising epistemological and cultural investment in quantitative measures such as randomized controlled trials and the advent of evidence-based medicine (EBM), the primary impetus behind biomedical research on CAM. In EBM, the evidence produced by clinical trials seems to speak for itself, divorced from human agency and social context. This evidence appears able to determine objectively, through numeric values, whether any given health intervention is safe and effective. As I argue below, however, EBM is also a strategy of professionalization not unlike other, more explicit profession-strengthening strategies employed in biomedicine over its history, such as regulatory limits on consultation with alternative practitioners and enforcement of laws of basic scientific literacy. Unlike these other strategies, however, evidence-based medicine can effect boundary work without seeming to do so at all.

Biomedicine's Shifting Terrain:
From Intuition and Experience to "Evidence"

Historically, the relative definitions of mainstream and alternative medicine have been fluid, their distinctions negotiated through processes that are decisively social and professionally motivated, even while they have been driven by concern for patient safety and health (R. Porter; Saks; Starr; Whorton).

Persuasion is a central element of that historical fluidity but the persuasive means through which those medical boundaries are established have shifted just as the ground upon which the health practices excluded from mainstream medicine has shifted.

In the eighteenth century, the US medical marketplace operated with a Wild-West mentality, with disparate groups of healers competing openly for patients. Protoprofessionalized practitioners, who were members of a guild and practiced outside of their homes, competed with midwives, bonesetters, and quacks for space in the medical ecosystem. Quacks—or "fakers and char-latans," as medical historian Roy Porter calls them—operated parasitically within that medical market, piggybacking on the success of the "regular" proto-professional practitioners of the time. Quacks were not antiestablishment: they did not subscribe to their own philosophical or therapeutic systems but rather sought to capitalize on the public's newfound thirst for medical goods. They traded on the esteem of the emerging medical profession by mimicking its modes of practice and its esoteric, technical language to attract customers in a market of competing healers.

By the 1800s, regular physicians saw their status rise dramatically as they ramped up efforts to organize themselves into a full-fledged profession, al-though these efforts were routinely challenged by a public that viewed healers of any kind with suspicion. Even some physicians resisted their colleagues' efforts to organize, particularly because ranks of physicians were at the time deeply divided by sectarianism. Some of these quarrels were fuelled by philo-sophical differences in their modes of practice; others, by turf wars in a com-petitive marketplace. During this period, regular physicians and sectarians such as homeopaths were often educated at the same institutions, although with different *materia medica* and clinical training.

Toward the end of the nineteenth century, regular physicians prevailed over sectarians as the dual forces of urbanization and science transformed the United States into a culture of expertise. The public relied ever more on the skills of professionals because, Starr notes, "the less one could believe 'one's own eyes'—and the new world of science continually prompted that feeling— the more receptive one became to seeing the world through the eyes of those who held specialized, technical knowledge, validated by communities of their peers" (19). Unlike the quacks of the eighteenth century, practitioners of "ir-regular" therapeutic systems such as homeopathy, naturopathy, Thomsonian-ism (medical botany), and mesmerism did take an explicitly antiestablishment approach as regular physicians achieved dominance over a narrowed market. Rather than try to align themselves with the fledgling medical profession, these practitioners set themselves in direct opposition to it. As Porter writes, "if this [new movement of irregular practitioners] was quackery, it was quackery with a difference" because the tone of the debate about medicine's boundaries had shifted from terms of the market to those of "ideology, philosophy, and morality" (*Quacks* 204). In response to these increasingly organized practitioners, the regular physicians strategically sought to preserve their newfound professional and epistemic territory. As I chronicle later in this chapter, their efforts to impede the activities of competing health practitioners through limitations on practice and demands for scientific literacy came ultimately to produce the medical profession as we know it today.

Sociologist Ayo Wahlberg extends Porter's analysis of eighteenth- and nineteenth-century tensions over medicine's boundaries to the late twentieth century, when "CAM" first emerged as a descriptive category. Wahlberg explains that, as public interest in CAM rose in the early 1990s, we were "once again witnessing the emergence of a quackery with a difference" (2315). Although this new phase of tension along the boundary between mainstream and alternative medicine was embedded within a long history of similar tensions, Wahlberg points out that the medical profession took a novel approach to protect its authority over matters of health: "Rather than ban or restrict access to CAM practitioners (as happened in the UK and many other countries in the early 20th century), the aim of contemporary efforts to regulate CAM has been recast into what might be termed a normalization of its practice and use" (2315).

Part of that normalization is the large-scale scientific testing of CAM. Calls for expanded biomedical research programs to investigate widespread interventions such as acupuncture, chiropractic, and herbal therapies came on the heels of Eisenberg and colleagues' game-changing survey of CAM use and expenditure published in the *New England Journal of Medicine* in 1993, which showed that far more Americans were using CAM than anyone in the medical community might have guessed. But the push to test CAM through scientific methods was also motivated by the larger shift toward evidence-based medicine (EBM) that took root in the 1990s, propelled by another groundbreaking article published just two months prior to the Eisenberg survey. In that article, from the November 4, 1992, issue of *JAMA*, a group of more than thirty medical researchers and practitioners advocated a new approach to patient care in which "best practice" would be determined not by the "intuition, unsystematic clinical experience, and pathophysiologic rationale" of individual doctors but by an empirical evidence base derived from clinical trials (Evidence-Based Medicine Working Group 2420). This new model of medical decision-making, EBM, was defined formally in a later article as "the conscientious, explicit, and judicious use of current best evidence in making decisions about the care of individual patients" (Sackett et al. 71). The emergence of EBM spurred the creation of vast research networks in all corners of medicine and crucially undergirded the push for the large-scale testing of CAM practices such as the studies published in the theme issues of *JAMA* and the *Archives*.

Only five years after the first article on EBM was published, the idea of EBM had taken root so vigorously that in 1997 physician-researchers Alvan Feinstein and Ralph Horwitz described it as having "acquired the kind of sanctity often accorded to motherhood, home, and the flag" (529). By the twelve year-mark, in 2004, sociologists Eric Mykhalovskiy and Lorna Weir observed more pointedly, in the words of their colleague, that "we live in a time of 'evidence-based everything'" (1060). Now, some twenty years after its entry into medical discourse, the phrase "evidence-based" has become such an unequivocal term of praise in contemporary culture that we currently count among the "evidence-based" health disciplines not only medicine and nursing but also dentistry, mental health, and occupational therapy. Beyond the sphere of medicine have developed a slew of evidence-based practices, including evidence-based communications, design, education, fitness, forestry, horsemanship, library and information practice, management, policy, scheduling, social work, and, within my own discipline, writing instruction.

The notion of evidence has by now been valorized to such an extent, in fact, that Cornell University currently hosts a blog entitled *Evidence-Based Living*, a clearinghouse dedicated to assessing "the scientific evidence on human problems and looking at how to use [that evidence] every day" ("About"). The blog's premise is that science (as a unitary cultural construct) not only *can* tell us how to make decisions and live our lives, but that it *should*—that it is a natural extension of scientific practice to weigh in on topics ranging from how to brush your teeth (the preferred method is the "Bass" technique but data are unclear), to making sure not to overbeat your scrambled eggs (otherwise the egg protein will uncoil too much and the eggs will become dry and tough), to whether or not a sports team can have too many star players (for football and basketball, yes; for baseball, no).[2]

Evidence is important because it tells us whether a given practice or procedure works so that we may direct our efforts, in whatever sphere of life, to those most likely to be effective. The move toward incorporating evidence into both medical and nonmedical domains signals collective efforts toward effectiveness and efficiency, a drive toward optimization that has flourished particularly under late capitalism. Evidence, in this context, provides a metric for determining the most productive course of action to achieve specifiable ends. However, as critics such as Feinstein and Horwitz and Mykhalovskiy and Weir point out, despite evidence-based medicine's wide influence both within medicine and beyond it, it is not without controversy.

In principle, EBM makes perfect sense: who would not want to practice (or receive) medicine that has been shown to work? But the paradigm of EBM precipitates intractable epistemic questions within biomedicine such as: What counts as "current best evidence"? Where does that evidence come from? Who judges it, and according to what criteria? EBM also raises significant concerns for the realm of practice: How ought one to proceed in the absence of evidence? Will EBM lead to an algorithmic or "cookbook" medicine? What becomes of clinical expertise and judgment? What was clinical medicine before it became "evidence-based"?[3]

The cultural weight assigned to the notion of evidence in medical discourse goes well beyond what evidence does in actual medical practice, extending into matters of power, prestige, and economic dominance. Medical historian George Weisz points out that, more than simply guiding best practice for doctors, evidence-based medicine serves as an important mechanism for "defending medical authority from a variety of contemporary threats," including insurance companies, patient demands, and alternative health practitioners (388). In other words, when the boundaries of biomedicine are up for negotiation, evidence-based medicine can help determine who belongs within those boundaries and who does not. In the case of biomedical research on complementary and alternative medicine, the limits of community membership are consequently shaped under the weight of available evidence.

Evidence-based medicine is often praised as the great leveler within the healthcare system. In 2001, for example, research methodologist Andrew J. Vickers argued that labels of "mainstream" and "alternative" are meaningless, that "what matters in EBM is evidence, not how a treatment is currently categorized" (1). More recently, Simon Singh and Edzard Ernst similarly asserted that evidence-based medicine "endorses any treatment that turns out to be effective, regardless of who is behind it, and regardless of how strange it might be" (26). For these commentators, and for others such as those whom I quoted at this chapter's outset (Fontanarosa and Lundberg of the *JAMA-Archives* theme issues and Angell and Kassirer of the *New England Journal of Medicine*), addressing the problem of CAM is simply a matter of putting CAM interventions to the test and then letting the evidence determine whether or not they are legitimate. Framing in this way the question of which CAM practices work and which do not, the individuals that perform the research appear simply to work in the service of the evidence they produce.

However, while the discourse of evidence-based medicine appeals to research values of objectivity and rigor, it is also a professionally interested discourse, one in which talk about "the evidence" is, in part, talk about jurisdictional control. Evidence reflects the character and limits of the communities that produce it.

Quantitative Evidence and Jurisdictional Control

Evidence in medicine is produced through research processes that appear to be divorced from human agency. Researchers design and report studies in ways that emphasize their adherence to scientific principles while deemphasizing their own perspectives as independent agents operating in a competitive and value-laden research culture. And yet, in even the most robustly designed and objective-seeming studies, "the language of science is seeded with social interest," as language and genre theorist Janet Giltrow has noted ("Modern Conscience" 173). Bearing traces of researchers' own subjectivities, attitudes, and values, medical journals therefore provide a window not only into procedures surrounding the production of knowledge but, more importantly for my purposes, into the dynamics of professional activity. Medical journals reflect the inherently competitive nature of what sociologist Andrew Abbott described as the professional ecosystem; examining the language of those journals shifts the debate about CAM research from terms that are strictly epistemological (i.e., that scientific methods will resolve the debate) toward those that are more explicitly social, even political.

In Abbott's view, professions are those occupations outside the commercial or industrial sphere whose main trade is in expertise. Their stores of abstract knowledge enable their control of other, related occupations because their abstract knowledge governs the practical knowledge necessary to performing the work. Abbott notes that "only a knowledge system governed by abstractions can redefine its problems and tasks, defend them from interlopers, and seize new problems. . . . Abstraction enables survival in the competitive system of professions" (9). According to Abbott, then, the professional landscape is not made up of a set of distinct, independent entities but, rather, is a system governed by tensions that continually reshape the relationships among them. The professions constitute an "interacting system" (33) within which competition is central: jurisdictional disputes arise necessarily when one profession claims territory formerly occupied by another. These disputes are part of the normal life of professions but, as Abbott points out, the more extensively and strongly organized professions tend to triumph over weaker ones.[4]

Professions are also inherently inegalitarian. As sociologist Paul Starr argued in 1982 in his landmark book *The Social Transformation of American Medicine*, each profession "claims to enjoy a dignity not shared by ordinary occupations and a right to set its own rules and standards" (37). In order to attain and maintain that position of privilege and its attendant autonomy and financial rewards, a profession must distinguish itself both from the public it serves and from other similar (and perhaps competing) occupational groups. The jurisdictional claim over CAM made in the *JAMA-Archives* illustrates Starr's point: by assuming the cultural and scientific authority to weigh in on a broad range of disparate health practices, the journals lay the medical profession's claim to jurisdiction already held by others, including CAM practitioners and, for self-administered therapies, members of the public.

Starr's view of the medical profession as inherently inegalitarian and antidemocratic resonates with more recent scholarship such as anthropologist Hans Baer's framing of the ascendance and maintenance of what he calls the "medical hegemony" of the United States as a site of capitalist struggle (35). Baer traces how different medical practices develop to reflect the diverse ideologies held by different segments of the population, concluding that individuals' use of various health systems (in various combinations) ultimately reflects their race, class, gender, and ethnicity. He argues that, as a result of capitalist influence, the biomedical paradigm—which eventually shaped all aspects of medical education, research, and practice—came to deflect the social origins of disease by emphasizing reactive intervention over proactive prevention. This emphasis, in Baer's view, shifted medicine toward a model of individualist care rather than of public health, thereby protecting the interests of the dominant class.[5]

Sociologist Mike Saks adopts a similar view of the medical profession, defining his project less in terms of capitalist dominance than in terms of the "politics of work." He argues that "successful occupations are seen as gaining increased income, status and power in the marketplace by socially excluding their competitors, who conversely lose out in the struggle for such rewards" (4). This process of exclusion depends in large part on defining CAM by what it is not, which is accomplished by gathering a range of disparate practices under a single rubric, "CAM," in which those practices are characterized principally by their political and professional marginality vis-à-vis biomedicine (e.g., their relative lack of research funding, exclusion from conventional medical curricula, denigration in medical journals, and tight regulations on their practice). As I illustrate in chapter 2, defining CAM as not-biomedicine is one of the primary rhetorical strategies through which the *JAMA-Archives* theme issues protect and maintain biomedicine's jurisdiction over CAM-related health practices.[6]

Professional dominance is always necessarily provisional, requiring constant maintenance with the competitive ecosystem of the professions. As Saks argues, "orthodox and alternative medicine are two seamlessly interrelated sides of the same coin" (162). The question of which health practices and practitioners end up on which side of that coin at any given time depends largely on what best serves the dominant profession's interest at that moment. Professions protect themselves against boundary incursion by situating their own expertise and modes of practice as the standard by which others ought to be measured. This strategy is evident in Fontanarosa and Lundberg's assertion I quoted at the start of this chapter, for instance—that "There is no alternative medicine. There is only scientifically proven, evidence-based medicine supported by solid data or unproven medicine, for which scientific evidence is lacking." One of the ways that the medical profession performs this protective work is through the discourse of quantification. Quantification abstracts numbers from the patients, practices, and practitioners they represent. By draining research knowledge of its personal and social interest, quantification can bolster authority, or even stand in for it, when professional boundaries are at stake.

Historian of science Theodore Porter refers to quantification as a "technology of distance" (ix). An eminently *social* technology, quantification plays a central role in biomedical boundary work because numbers seem to decouple knowledge from those who make it. By standardizing, counting, measuring, ranking, and comparing the objects of their research, researchers themselves, as individual subjects, recede from sight. Their studies no longer appear to represent a view from somewhere—that is, from the position of the researcher-subject—but rather a view from nowhere, an objective position (see Nagel). As rhetorician Jessica Mudry has observed, "Because pure objectivity lies at the heart of quantification, it claims to defy social and cultural constraints and immunity from sociological analysis or criticism" (135). Phrased even more simply, quantitative discourse persuades because numbers "don't lie." From this perspective, numbers instead seem to sit naked, ready for re-numeration by different observers on different calculators, promising they will remain true.

While knowledge-makers are subject to the fits and fashions of a given research culture, numbers, seemingly divorced from human agency, appear to hold tight in their significations. This is why Theodore Porter distinguishes between what Allan Megill has referred to as *disciplinary objectivity*, an objectivity produced through expert consensus (Megill 5), and what Porter terms *mechanical objectivity*, the objectivity produced by numbers. Unlike disciplinary objectivity, which is contingent and developed through complex negotiation, mechanical objectivity consists in rules and procedures that aim to "make it impossible for personal biases or preferences to affect the outcome of an investigation" (T. Porter 4). Procedures in medical research such as standardization, blind assessment, and statistical analysis, for instance, attempt to filter out a researcher's own hunches or preferences by using methods that are, in a sense, bigger than any one individual. When variables are standardized, they are rendered similar enough to be compared; when researchers are unaware of whether a participant received an active treatment or placebo, they see in their assessment of the intervention what is there to see, rather than what they want to see; when data are analyzed mathematically for statistical prevalence and patterns, their significance is determined by a set of numbers, not a person.

The numbers produced in biomedical research are emptied of their social interest through their method of production, the randomized controlled trial (RCT), which transforms a variable range of health problems, treatments, practitioners, and patients into measurable phenomena by operating in accordance within a set of rigid criteria and procedures. This transformation of people, practices, and effects into measurable phenomena allows us to compare "disparate objects" according to a shared metric (Mudry 42). This means that, in research on CAM, quantification would ideally allow researchers to calculate and compare the effects of disparate treatments such as pills and acupuncture needles to determine which, if either, is most effective for treating a predefined condition. The question of whether or not a given alternative health practice "works" is (or, rather, appears to be) divested of personal or professional interest as it is translated into a numeric value that can be compared and ranked against conventional medical treatments.

Although numbers produced in biomedical research signify constancy and calculability, Thomas Gieryn reminds us that, in the cultural maintenance of scientific boundaries, the relationship between science and numbers is better understood as "contingent, variously made or severed as players— 'scientific' or not—assign or deny credibility to claims" (*Cultural Boundaries* 189n17). That is, it is not just *that* numbers are used in a given effort to create impartial, reliable knowledge; it is *how* those numbers are used and by *whom*. It is significant, then, that both the call for expanded data on CAM's safety and efficacy and the answer to that call in the form of clinical trials originated within biomedicine itself. CAM practitioners generally do not rely on trial evidence in their practice (Villanueva-Russell), and most CAM patients use CAM regardless of whether or not scientific evidence supports the therapy in question (Astin).

When biomedical boundaries are up for negotiation, the context and purpose of quantitative research data are therefore often as important as the data themselves. CAM practices are typically understood in North America in opposition to, and often as incompatible with, biomedicine. Practices such as traditional Chinese medicine, chiropractic, and naturopathy are generally administered by practitioners who do not hold conventional medical credentials (i.e., degrees in medicine, nursing, or allied health professions). Part of the allure of such practices, to many, is precisely their status as alternatives to mainstream medicine, particularly for those with chronic or ambiguous conditions or for those who seek care through what they believe to be a more humanized, holistic approach to health. For such individuals, the system out of which a given health intervention emerges is often as important as the intervention itself. For example, while spinal manipulation is the central intervention in chiropractic care, chiropractors also actively engage the psychosocial dimensions of care through techniques such as affective talk and touching.[7] It is difficult to isolate manipulation from these "softer" aspects of chiropractic, and any attempt to deliver manipulation without them could well eliminate the same elements of the practice that so many individuals find appealing (and, it should be said, effective) about chiropractic. Even still, RCTs of CAM practices generally only test the central intervention, such as spinal manipulation, rather than the practice as a whole, fundamentally distorting the very practices they investigate. In such cases, negative trial results are often attributed to the ineffectiveness of the interventions studied rather than to failures of trial design to capture any potential effectiveness. (I examine such issues at length in chapters 3 and 4.)

In the view of the editors of the coordinated theme issues of *JAMA* and the *Archives*, the thirteen RCT reports published within the journals nevertheless provided depth to an otherwise shallow evidence base on CAM. Four of these clinical trials evaluated orally administered herbal supplements, three evaluated acupuncture and acupuncture-related interventions, and the remainder evaluated chiropractic, topical lanolin, yoga, aromatherapy, relaxation exercises, and homeopathy.[8] Five of the interventions studied were found to be at least partly effective, including Chinese herbal medicine for irritable bowel syndrome (Bensoussan et al.), lanolin and breast shields for nursing women (Brent et al.), traditional Chinese medicine for breech pregnancies (Cardini and Weixin), yoga for carpal tunnel syndrome (Garfinkel et al.), and aromatherapy for alopecia areata (Hay, Jamieson, and Ormerod). The remaining interventions were found to have little or no effect. All of the primary authors were biomedically trained, most with MD and/or PhD degrees, while only two trials were conducted by coresearchers with CAM credentials.[9]

The authors of these studies generally align themselves with the values of evidence-based medicine by acknowledging their adherence to methods that are the hallmark of EBM, such as blinding, randomization, and statistical analysis. In doing so, these researchers assert their status as medical insiders despite their work on "outsider" interventions. For instance, in the theme issue of *Archives of Dermatology*, Hay, Jamieson, and Omerod report on their RCT for aromatherapy as a treatment for alopecia areata, emphasizing not only their study's strong positive finding of the treatment's effectiveness but also that their study "successfully applied an evidence-based method to an alternative therapy" (1349).

Some critics within the *JAMA-Archives* theme issues draw on the framework of evidence-based medicine to explain the lack of quantitative evidence on CAM as due to faults in the practices themselves. Tom Delbanco, for instance, argues in his *JAMA* editorial that clinical trials of CAM are a waste of time and resources because any apparent effectiveness of CAM is due to nothing more than a placebo effect. In his view, CAM practitioners manipulate their patients with "primal message[s] of hope" to encourage frequent, and lucrative, visits (1560).

Others, such as James Dalen, the editor of *Archives of Internal Medicine*, offer a more even-tempered view of the evidence base for CAM, arguing in his theme issue editorial that we ought not to judge CAM unnecessarily harshly, lest biomedicine be held to the same standards of evidence. Identifying himself as an adherent of EBM, Dalen methodically dismantles the argument that CAM is unscientific because it lacks a substantial evidence base. Pointing to gaps in evidence regarding frontline interventions for cardiovascular diseases, Dalen argues that if acupuncture, chiropractic, and herbal remedies are deemed unscientific due to poor evidence, then so too should be aspirin, warfarin, and heparin, which were introduced as antithrombotic agents before the dawn of the RCT, as well as bedside pulmonary artery catheterization, which had been performed since 1970 without any trial evidence supporting its use.

Critiquing the medical profession's efforts to buttress its boundaries, Dalen's own conclusion is that "the principal distinguishing characteristic of unconventional and conventional medicine therapies is their source of introduction. Conventional therapies are introduced by mainstream Western physicians and scientists, whereas most unconventional modalities are introduced by 'outsiders'" (2180). As I explain in the section that follows, this language of "insiders" and "outsiders" runs through the history of the medical profession in the United States. The profession's rise to prominence over the nineteenth century depended on that tension between insiders and outsiders as various practitioners jostled for jurisdiction over matters of health. However, the emergence of quantitative research methodologies in the mid-twentieth century transferred from the medical profession to the notion of evidence itself the authority to determine which health practices and practitioners were in and which were out.

Medical-Professional Strategies of Exclusion

To consider evidence-based medicine more fully in its capacity as a profession-defining measure rather than simply as a neutral model of evidence production and clinical decision-making, I now turn briefly to two of its historical antecedents, the American Medical Association's consultation clause and the enactment of state-level basic science laws. These measures were ostensibly adopted in the service of patients, but they were rooted also in concerns about preserving professional jurisdiction. Below, I situate the episode of boundary work precipitated by the *JAMA-Archives* theme issues on CAM within the context of these earlier episodes both to highlight its lineage in the ongoing process of boundary work and to illustrate how this most recent episode stands apart for its invocation of quantitative evidence as the touchstone of legitimacy in health care. Although the editors of *JAMA* and the *Archives* assert that new and better evidence will answer our questions about CAM once and for all, other exigencies for boundary work will always inevitably follow—such exigencies are a part of the normal life of the professions.

When the American Medical Association (AMA) was founded in 1847, one of its goals was to give physicians greater control over their profession and edge out competition in an otherwise unregulated medical marketplace. One of its initial legislative acts was to adopt the now-infamous consultation clause within its code of ethics. This clause aimed to prevent members from associating in any professional context with outside practitioners: "no one can be considered as a regular practitioner, or a fit associate in consultation, whose practice is based upon an exclusive dogma, to the rejection of the accumulated experience of the profession" (qtd. in Whorton, *Nature Cures* 69). Such exclusionary provisions had been immensely successful in the United Kingdom, where practitioners feared ostracism if they consulted with irregulars. In one extreme case, for example, when former British Prime Minister Benjamin Disraeli fell gravely ill in 1881, he was treated by a homeopath until his aides entreated Richard Quain, a specialist in bronchial disorders, to examine him. Quain refused the request, however, claiming that the College of Physicians would expel him for practicing alongside an irregular. He only agreed to treat Disraeli at Queen Victoria's command. Despite the queen's orders, Quain's acquiescence ignited a long political and professional debate within the college in the months after Disraeli's death.[10]

The consultation clause did not have as powerful an effect in the United States. While restrictions on consultation appealed to Britain's richly stratified society, the United States' populist leanings aligned public sympathy with the irregulars—and with patients' right to choose among practitioners. The clause was therefore difficult to enforce and by 1903, its support within the profession had withered. An "advisory document" took its place, which discredited irregular practices but stipulated that physicians must consult with whomever necessary to serve their patients' best interests. Prohibitions on consultation with irregulars nevertheless remained one of the few tools available to the AMA to restrict competition, and similar bans were enforced against osteopaths in 1938 and chiropractors in the 1960s, the latter ban resulting in a protracted but eventually successful antitrust lawsuit against the AMA and codefendants by five chiropractors, launched in 1976 and concluded in 1992.[11]

The enactment of independent basic science laws across twenty-three states between 1925 and 1979 also sought to weed competing practitioners out of the health care market. These laws required health care practitioners to demonstrate basic knowledge of the biological sciences prior to licensure. On the surface, these laws served to protect patients by ensuring that all health practitioners, including CAM practitioners, held enough basic scientific literacy and understanding of bodily processes to care effectively for patients. However, according to medical historian Norman Gevitz, these laws were intended primarily as a form of gatekeeping, with the presumption that unconventional health practitioners would not be able to pass the basic science examinations. But the exams had unintended consequences: up to a third of United States-trained MDs and over half of foreign-trained MDs also failed them (Gevitz 59). Given the high failure rate of even conventional physicians, it is no surprise that the basic science laws were progressively repealed between 1967 and 1979, when the last law was struck down. As with the AMA's consultation clause, the basic science requirements may ultimately have backfired on regular medicine: as Whorton notes, instead of forcing unconventional practitioners to abandon the health care field, the laws "forc[ed] irregulars to sink or swim. They chose to swim, and that meant they had to elevate the level of instruction they provided their students in medical science" ("Cultism to CAM" 232).

Both of these exclusionary measures, the consultation clause and basic science laws, sought to differentiate practitioners of mainstream medicine from those who did not share the profession's allegiance to scientific values. The irony, of course, is that these measures may have inadvertently spurred alternative practitioners to organize themselves in order to meet the scientific demands placed on them. What is most significant about the medical profession's efforts to enact such exclusionary measures, then, is not that they provide evidence of medicine's basis in science but, rather, that such measures bespeak the profession's fundamental insecurity about its own jurisdiction over matters of health and illness by trying to weed out competing practitioners. In the consultation clause, that insecurity operated in disguise as concern for patients, while in the basic science laws, its disguise was concern about scientific literacy.

The rise of the randomized controlled trial within biomedicine followed a similar trajectory: appeals for evidence on individual health practices were framed as concern for patient health and safety but were no less motivated by professional concern. As Theodore Porter notes, quantitative measures such as RCTs "work mainly as social technologies, not guides to private thinking" (208). As a "technology of trust" (Porter's term), the RCT holds a nearly sacred status in evidence-based medicine, its aura cast so widely that it has come to seem both natural and inevitable as a research methodology. However, the RCT first emerged in the 1940s and 1950s not in medicine but in the agricultural and statistical sciences, only gaining gradual acceptance in medicine over the decades that followed (Devereaux and Yusuf; T. Porter). The fabled first biomedical RCT was the 1948 British Medical Research Council trial of streptomycin for pulmonary tuberculosis, which, along with other trials of the period, enacted a fledgling methodology that applied a laboratory model to clinical research; this laboratory model promised to minimize bias and the effects of chance in evaluating medical treatments. The goal of the RCT method was to produce a body of data on specified health interventions that could be quantified through statistical analysis, providing researchers with accurate and reliable results.[12]

The push for quantitative methods in medicine did not come from practitioners, who generally resisted the idea of standardized models of care, viewing such standardization as a machination of legislators to curb their clinical authority. Instead, the initial push for quantification came from regulatory authorities who sought to establish "uniform and rigorous standards" of practice and so viewed physicians' expertise, rooted in experience, as "a valuable and dangerous commodity" (T. Porter 206). Midcentury policy changes also helped advance acceptance of the RCT in the United States, particularly through two acts of Congress that expanded the regulatory purview of the Food and Drug Administration (FDA). The first legislative act, the Federal Food, Drug, and Cosmetic Act of 1938, gave the relatively toothless FDA power to reject drugs deemed dangerous, although it was not authorized to make determinations of efficacy. One result of this limitation was that many drugs on the market, though proven safe, had no real effect. As Porter points out, however, the FDA sometimes circumvented this proscription against determining efficacy by rejecting inert drugs as dangerous on the grounds that they could be used in the place of effective ones.

While the experience of individual clinicians remained important to the FDA in its drug evaluations even after the 1938 Act, the research scene changed dramatically with the passing of the Kefauver-Harris Bill in 1962. Prompted by the thalidomide scandal, the bill mandated that drugs be proved not only safe but also effective, finally edging out clinical expertise and positioning the RCT as the ideal form of evaluation. Since that time, the emphasis in medical research has shifted from small RCTs with sensitive outcomes assessment (e.g., patient self-reports, pain assessment scales) toward large-scale RCTs that focus primarily on "major clinical outcomes (e.g., death, stroke)" (Devereaux and Yusuf 106). These shifts in outcomes measures reflect an overall shift in medicine toward ever cruder estimates of health and illness wherein, as Ted Kaptchuk argues, research becomes less about "emphasizing outcomes" than about "the purity of the means" of obtaining them ("Powerful" 1724).

Shifting the question of *what* we know in medicine to *how* we know it, Kaptchuk explains, the randomized controlled trial has thus come to be seen, both within the scientific community and beyond, as "medicine's most reliable method for 'representing things as they really are' " ("Double-Blind" 541). Yet the significance of the RCT in evidence production in medicine can easily be overestimated, largely because of how high the RCT sits, hierarchically, over other research methods such as unblinded studies or case reports. This overestimation is particularly true in debates about complementary and alternative medicine, where the "best available evidence" (Sackett et al.) comes to mean almost exclusively evidence derived from RCTs, despite the insistence of the original advocates of EBM that the highest-level *available* evidence at any time is grounds enough for evidence-based practice, even if it is derived from observational or case studies.

In their ideal form, once exclusion criteria have been applied, RCTs randomly divide experimental participants into groups that receive the therapy under study ("intervention" groups) and groups that do not ("control" groups).

All participants in the intervention group receive the same treatment, regardless of their individual health history or concomitant conditions. Participants across both groups are matched to some extent for age, sex, and other characteristics that triallists deem necessary. Participants are usually blinded to their intervention assignment as a precaution against placebo effects, which occur when participants in the control group experience improvement despite having received only an inert simulation of the study intervention. Researchers are also usually blinded to avoid bias as they evaluate outcomes and to prevent them from unintentionally communicating cues to participants regarding intervention assignments. (For more on RCT design, see Jadad and Enkin.)

Studies of complementary and alternative medicine pose significant methodological problems because the practices do not translate easily into the "gold standard" RCT format. Randomization and standardization are foreign concepts in health practices such as traditional Chinese medicine and chiropractic, and are often incommensurate with them. In contrast to biomedicine, these practices view patients as fundamentally unique, so two people with the same ailment might be treated altogether differently, depending on their unique constellation of symptoms and personal characteristics, such as height, weight, temperament, allergies, and health history (Barry 2647; Degele 118). This emphasis on uniqueness means that treatments can be difficult to standardize in experimental settings: while biomedical treatment is largely symptomatic in the sense that a person may be treated separately for different complaints (even by separate specialists)—one pill for headache, say, another for constipation, and another still for irritability (these are Degele's examples; 118)—CAM practitioners such as chiropractors and TCM practitioners typically aim to address all symptoms together.[13]

Controlling and blinding studies of manual practices such as acupuncture and chiropractic are also problematic because their therapies include unmistakable physical actions that are difficult to simulate, such as piercing the skin with a steel needle and moving the spine with an often audible popping sound. Pharmaceutical trials are usually easy to control and blind by substituting the active drug with a lookalike sugar pill, or placebo. Once participants have been assigned to treatment or control groups, no one but the study's pharmacist need know to which group any participant is assigned because all participants will receive interventions that appear to be the same. Controlling a practice such as acupuncture is more difficult because there is no available control that is both realistic and definitely inert (à la sugar pill), and practitioners usually cannot be blinded. These methodological problems leave researchers to puzzle out how such studies ought to be conducted, interpreted, and incorporated into practice. The question for biomedical researchers of how to proceed with testing CAM in an evidence-based framework is nested in a complex web of factors—disciplinary, professional, epistemic, generic, philosophical, commercial, and regulatory.

For the clinical trials published in the theme issues of *JAMA* and the *Archives*, the stringency of their methods, including their randomization, blinding, and use of placebo controls, correlates with the study interventions' modes of delivery: trials of interventions that can be administered somewhat like pharmaceuticals, such as aromatherapy and herbal supplements, are randomized, double-blinded, and placebo-controlled; while those that require practitioners and/or participants to engage in specific behaviors that vary by group assignment, such as acupuncture, chiropractic, relaxation exercises, and yoga, feature only partial blinding and limited use of controls. In all cases, treatments were standardized even though, in practice, most of the interventions under study would be administered differently to different patients with the same conditions, as I described above. Although all of the trials published in the theme issues utilized two or more intervention arms (minimally, control and intervention arms) and ran various statistical analyses on the data, the trial populations were fairly small, ranging from 30 to 302 participants, with a mean of 116 participants and a median of 76. The reliability and statistical power of these studies may therefore potentially limit the generalizability of their results.

Once trial data have been produced, however problematically, another issue that affects the evidence base on individual CAM interventions is that the data are aggregated in systematic reviews, such as those of the Cochrane Collaboration, and in clinical practice guidelines. The Cochrane Collaboration is a worldwide network of volunteers that produce and publish systematic reviews on all manner of health topics; each review evaluates the current state of evidence and makes recommendations for practice based on available data. These aggregative methods reify the RCT-derived data, producing metadata that is constituted as the firm ground upon which clinical recommendations are made within the EBM framework. As Ezzo and colleagues discuss in the *JAMA* theme issue, however, limitations on the quantity and quality of data on CAM can skew evidence within the Cochrane Collaboration against interventions that may, in practice, have higher levels of safety and efficacy than trial data show. The authors cite several factors that limit the comprehensiveness of such reviews, such as publication bias, which they argue might result in disproportionately high rates of publication of CAM studies with negative findings as compared to biomedical studies with negative findings.

A further problem with availability of RCT-derived evidence on CAM is simply that it is difficult to come by, with trials relatively rare since they are difficult to fund without industry-based sponsors. Persistent public funding shortages negatively affect medical research generally because funding from pharmaceutical companies has become so integral that many important studies of older, off-patent drugs and newer, nonblockbuster drugs are simply not being conducted (Angell; Held, Wedel, and Wilhelmsen). This is all the more true of studies of CAM, which offer relatively little patent control or profit potential.

Given such limitations on the quantity and quality of RCT evidence on CAM (and there are more, as I show in later chapters), CAM is vulnerable to the call in biomedicine to reject practices lacking "solid evidence." This vulnerability can be used to shift boundary lines in biomedicine's favor. The invocation of evidence-based medicine can therefore function in biomedical discourse about CAM as an exclusionary measure on the same order as the consultation clause and basic science laws. All of these measures were adopted in the name of medical science and patient care, but each has simultaneously served the interests of the medical profession. In the CAM-themed issues of *JAMA* and the *Archives*, evidence-based medicine is constructed as the point-of-access on the biomedical border: *JAMA*'s editors suggest that any intervention can get in provided that it has evidence to support its entry. But in its reliance on quantification as a technology of distance, evidence-based medicine glosses over the role that members of the medical profession play, wittingly or not, as attendants at the gate.[14]

*

As I have shown in this chapter, the first serious, concerted efforts to establish an evidence base for alternative health practices began more than two decades ago, and yet the terms of the debate about which practices are legitimate and which are not remain substantially the same today. In September 2014, for instance, sixteen years following the publication of the *JAMA-Archives* theme issues, the website of the magazine the *Atlantic* featured an article by James Hamblin with a title that nods directly toward Fontanarosa and Lundberg's *JAMA* editorial in 1998. In Hamblin's article, "There is no 'Alternative Medicine,'" he reports on the fallout of a large, multicenter, randomized controlled trial of chelation therapy for heart disease published in *JAMA* the previous spring.[15] Chelation therapy, an intravenous intervention for removal of heavy metals from the bloodstream, is rarely used in biomedicine, usually only in cases of acute lead or other metal poisonings. In such cases, fluids such as ethylenediaminetetraacetic acid (EDTA) are injected to form molecular bonds with the metals that then together pass through the kidneys and out of the body in the urine. Outside of biomedicine, chelation therapy is used much more widely, usually by CAM practitioners, ostensibly to treat a range of symptoms and conditions that include arthritis, hormonal disorders, and heart disease. A naturopathic clinic near my own house in Toronto offers chelation therapy among a range of other modalities that include botanical medicine, homeopathy, nutritional therapy, naturopathic manipulation, electro-interstitial scanning, and intravenous and intramuscular therapies. In his *Atlantic* article, Hamblin, a trained physician, estimates that some 100,000 "sick, desperate, and uninformed or misinformed" Americans seek chelation therapy from CAM practitioners each year.

The controversy that Hamblin cites erupted following the publication of a study in *JAMA* by Lamas and colleagues in March 2013 that compared disodium EDTA chelation therapy to placebo in participants with heart disease. This clinical trial found a slight but statistically significant positive effect in the total reduction of morbidity and morality in the chelation group. Alongside this study, *JAMA* published a searing critique of its reliability by Steven Nissen, chair of cardiology at the Cleveland Clinic. Nissen's article advances a set of arguments about well-designed randomized controlled trials in the production of evidence that were, by 2013, well established in the medical community; I examined some such arguments above and take up more in later chapters.

What I want to highlight here is Hamblin's own coverage of the *JAMA* blow-up about chelation therapy because it reveals that debates regarding CAM's place in biomedicine were no more settled in 2014 than they were in 1998. Adopting a line of thinking that has now become familiar, Hamblin writes: "'Alternative medicine' is itself a strange notion, in that there are really only three kinds of medicine: medicine that is proven to work, medicine that is proven not to work, and medicine that has not been conclusively studied." Hamblin's concern in this article about the safety and welfare (and wallets) of the American public regarding CAM is certainly justified: people have the right to know whether or not the health products or services they consume will help and not hurt them, and rigorous scientific testing, despite the problems it poses, is the only way to determine that. Further, there is an intuitive appeal to Hamblin's assertion, like those of earlier commentators, that enough evidence of a given CAM intervention's effect can and will ensure its acceptance into biomedicine. However, as appealing as this assertion is, I show in the remaining chapters that the concept of evidence within contemporary biomedicine is slipperier and more elastic than any of these authors allow. It is elastic enough, in fact, that it can be called upon to draw boundary lines of various sorts, expanding, contracting, or reinforcing the borders of what counts as safe, effective health care.

In *Cultural Boundaries of Science*, Thomas Gieryn identifies his motivation as "to make the science wars historically mundane by showing that they are of a piece with [previous] episodes of cultural cartography" of science (337). As this chapter has demonstrated, recent efforts to define the boundaries between mainstream and alternative medicine are, in a sense, "of a piece" with previous moments of boundary work in the history of medicine—they are mundane, just part of the normal evolution of biomedical science as both a profession and a bounded cultural space. However, what distinguishes the debates about CAM that began in the early 1990s from those that came before is that they are premised on a qualitatively new understanding of evidence and how evidence ought to be produced and applied. Hamblin's core argument, for example, is identical to those of Fontanarosa and Lundberg and Angell and Kassirer from 1998, that evidence alone will decide the worth of CAM. Importantly, however, under the framework of evidence-based medicine, the threshold of what counts as evidence for CAM seems to be even higher than for mainstream biomedical interventions (Borgerson; Morreim). Over the remainder of this book, I explain how these standards are invoked within the *JAMA-Archives* theme issues and their surrounding medical-professional and public discourse to strengthen and expand the boundaries of biomedicine.

Patrolling Professional Borders

The key argument on which debates about complementary and alternative medicine (CAM) generally turn is whether CAM is scientific, or even can be. We saw this argument in the previous chapter in the editors' introduction to the 1998 coordinated theme issues of the journals of the American Medical Association: "There is no alternative medicine. There is only scientifically proven, evidence-based medicine supported by solid data or unproven medicine, for which scientific evidence is lacking" (Fontanarosa and Lundberg, "Alternative Medicine" 1618). We saw this, too, in similar arguments from Angell and Kassirer in the *New England Journal of Medicine* and from physician James Hamblin in the *Atlantic*.

Even the charismatic astrophysicist and giant of popular science Neil deGrasse Tyson has weighed in on the debate, posting a joke on Twitter in May 2012 that has since been retweeted more than 3,600 times and favorited by almost a thousand people: "Q: What do you call Alternative Medicine that survives double-blind laboratory tests? A: Regular Medicine." This joke feels instantly familiar because, like other arguments that "there is no alternative medicine," it is premised on a specific understanding of biomedical evidence production, which holds that research on any health intervention proceeds straightforwardly, without interest, from the identification of research questions through to study design and execution to data analysis. In this view of research, data are ratified as "evidence" only on their publication within peer-reviewed journals, which then ultimately form the ground upon which medical providers and legislators base future policy and practice. This is the ideal of research, certainly, but it underemphasizes a key element of the research process: the production of evidence in medicine is an eminently social process.

One of the most generative premises of science studies over the past five decades is that science both produces and is produced by communities of scientists. The pervasive public representation of the scientist as a "lone genius" (Charney)—one whose skilled, dispassionate application of scientific principles to complex phenomena is punctuated by flashes of individual brilliance—has been dispelled by scholars investigating the social dimensions of scientific activity both upstream in laboratory work and academic publication and downstream in policymaking and popular media.[1] As Thomas Kuhn articulated half a century ago in his game-changing book *The Structure of Scientific Revolutions*, the work of science is rooted not in scientists' individual practice or objective knowledge but in their collective efforts toward building consensus about what we know about the world and how it works.

Rhetoric is central to Kuhn's model of scientific change: members of scientific communities can be "persuaded to change their minds" (152); they are subject to "transformations of vision" (111) and "conversion" (204); and they experience shifts in their "professional allegiances" (158)—all of which are the product of community activity. So effective are scientific communities' efforts at consensual knowledge-making that these communal efforts are virtually invisible within the robust knowledge they produce. But it is only on the surface that scientific knowledge is independent of those that produce it. As this chapter illustrates, the social dimensions of science are all the more significant when its boundaries are up for negotiation.

In considering how the notion of evidence determines the boundaries of biomedicine, peer-reviewed journals offer a window into the sociality of science. As Charles Bazerman and James Paradis argued in their now-canonical collection *Textual Dynamics of the Professions*, examining the bidirectional relationship between a profession and its texts can illuminate the roles those professions play in the drama of social life: "Out of provisional clusterings of people, activities, and language emerge highly organized professions of great social consequence. Once established, professions maintain their organization, power, and activity in large part through networks of texts. As these professions increasingly form the framework of modern existence, their texts set the terms of our lives" (4). Taking my cue from Bazerman and Paradis, I examine in this chapter how the contributors to the CAM-themed issues of *JAMA* and the *Archives* situate their texts, on subjects not typically under the purview of such journals, in relation to the historical-professional dynamics that have shaped biomedicine. Predictably, most of the contributors to the journals frame the tension between mainstream and alternative medicine as the demarcation of practices that are scientific from those that are not. Such an account places CAM on the fringes of North American health care because of its lack of scientific rigor. However, as the previous chapter explained, the boundary between mainstream and alternative medicine ought to be understood, equally, as a boundary between dominant and marginal systems of knowledge and practice.

In what follows, I demonstrate that biomedicine is bounded, in part, by how medical researchers and practitioners define and categorize the practices that comprise CAM. My fundamental claim is that the *JAMA-Archives* theme issues on CAM, as a set of texts curated by the publication arm of a professional medical association, preserve biomedicine's historical coherence as a firmly defined discipline while simultaneously stretching its limits to reach practices formerly beyond its scope. This process appears to serve inherently epideictic functions, reinforcing both conventional biomedical community values and the apparent boundaries separating health professions even as some community members seek ostensibly to eradicate those boundaries.[2]

I begin the chapter by examining the coordinated CAM-themed issues of *JAMA* and the *Archives* in the context of professional discourse as constitutive of the professions that engage in it. In responding to the journals' call for papers, the contributors identify themselves as members of a community that only came into being with the publication of the journals themselves. Admission within the boundaries of this community is determined partly by the processes of editorial selection and peer review, which I argue in the second section function, in part, as strategies of professional self-regulation.

In the remaining two sections, I examine the various definitions and historical descriptions of CAM offered by contributors to the *JAMA-Archives* theme issues. These accounts aggregate together health practices as diverse as chiropractic, energy healing, herbal medicine, massage therapy, and prayer under a single umbrella category whose sole organizing logic is that its contents do not count as medicine. As others have noted, this aggregative process functionally redefines CAM practices in the negative, as "not-biomedicine." Within the *JAMA-Archives* theme issues, this negative categorization—what Bowker and Star call a "residual category"—conceals the historical and theoretical foundations of individual CAM modalities, redefining them instead, as a collective, in biomedical terms. These redefined, biomedicalized CAM practices are then operationalized in clinical trials, but the practices as they appear in those studies often bear little resemblance to the practices as they occur in their native contexts of use.

From a functional perspective, of course, biomedical researchers must redefine CAM practices to some extent within biomedical terms simply to do their work: most of the practices that comprise CAM are, on their own terms, incompatible with standard scientific procedures. However, one of the rhetorical outcomes of redefining a range of diverse alternative health practices as an aggregated collective, "CAM," is that the process likewise redefines the criteria for determining whether a given intervention counts as legitimate and effective or not. For example, many CAM interventions are individualized for specific patients (Barry 2647; Degele 118) but are standardized when molded into a medical-scientific framework, consequently requiring that intervention to perform equally across populations rather than to show effectiveness in individual bodies. In the original CAM practice, however, that individualization may be exactly what makes the intervention seem effective to the person using it.

Examining how the *JAMA-Archives* theme issues on CAM constitute the medical profession and redefine the CAM practices over which it claims jurisdiction illustrates how peer-reviewed scientific publications actively, though not necessarily consciously, regulate medical-professional borders. By tracking points of disjunction between CAM interventions as they are defined in medical journals and their enactment in practice, we can see more clearly how, in CAM research, the deck may be stacked against the interventions under study. One of chief reasons that biomedical boundary work is so effective at preserving biomedicine's cultural and epistemic authority, I argue, is that it reifies the boundaries it produces. In the *JAMA-Archives* theme issues, the contributors' explicit and self-conscious efforts at defining their profession's borders are seamless, almost invisible. Instead of foregrounding the fluidity of professional boundaries, they naturalize them, rendering them more stable, not less.

Constituting the Medical Profession

In December 1997, when Phil Fontanarosa and George Lundberg issued their call for papers for the CAM-themed issues of *JAMA* and the *Archives*, they called forth a community of scholars that did not exist prior to the call itself. Biomedical researchers had of course published on interventions such as chiropractic and acupuncture before 1998.[3] However, that previous research appeared in isolated articles across both mainstream and alternative medical journals, whereas, Fontanarosa and Lundberg argued, their theme issues would be different:

The 1998 coordinated theme issues will provide a unique, multidisciplinary forum for the publication of original research studies and scholarly articles that present new scientific information and innovative ideas on complementary and alternative medicine to the medical and scientific community. By stimulating research and giving emphasis to this topic, we hope to promote widespread attention in the medical literature and the lay media, foster education among health care professionals, and increase knowledge among patients and the public. ("Call for Papers" 2111–12)

Fontanarosa and Lundberg assured potential contributors that all submissions would be "subject to our usual rigorous editorial evaluation and peer review" (2112), an assurance that indicates their belief that accepted submissions would be admitted into their profession's store of knowledge, on a par with more conventional research.

The following November, Fontanarosa and Lundberg specified more clearly in the theme issue of *JAMA* that the theme issues were distinct from previous publications on CAM in their meta-turn, their self-consciousness as "a planned, concerted effort" to compile scholarship on CAM from an explicitly biomedical perspective ("Alternative Medicine" 1618). In the editors' view, this concerted assessment of CAM within a biomedical context was a first for the medical profession. Certainly, this is true, but more significant is that the journals addressed the biomedical community as though research on CAM were already under biomedicine's official purview, even though, as the editors themselves argued, the theme issues on CAM represented a sea-change for the medical profession. From a rhetorical perspective, this mode of address is significant because, in framing CAM research as uncontroversial, the journals are prescriptive rather than descriptive: they aim not to reflect the current state of medical research but to shape it. The *JAMA-Archives* coordinated theme issues are therefore an instance of what Maurice Charland defines as constitutive rhetoric, a rhetoric in which subjects are constituted by the very discourses with which they are addressed.[4]

Charland mobilizes Kenneth Burke's notion of identification and Louis Althusser's notion of interpellation to show that individuals are constructed as subjects discursively, a subjectivity that they then affirm as they engage in action in the social world.[5] I trace this constitutive process in the *JAMA-Archives* in the context of professional discourse, examining the role of editorial evaluation and peer review as gatekeeping mechanisms. Although peer evaluation is central to the validation of knowledge claims in research culture, these practices may threaten the very values they appear to preserve, such as communalism and objectivity. The community that is subsequently brought into being through peer review in the *JAMA-Archives* is necessarily founded on an awareness of, and struggle over, professional boundaries.

According to Charland, interpellation "occurs at the very moment one enters into a rhetorical situation, that is, as soon as an individual recognizes and

acknowledges being addressed" (220). Although Charland was writing specifically in a political/policy context, his model of constitutive rhetoric can usefully be brought to bear on health and medicine, as Judy Segal has done on the
construction of the headache patient as a rhetorical audience in the clinical exchange (*Health*). For the *JAMA-Archives* theme issues, Charland's framework
shifts the set of questions we might imagine being asked and answered within
the journals. Instead of asking, for example, *whether* a legitimate, biomedical
community of CAM researchers exists, the journals seem instead to ask *where*
that community can be found. (The journals' seeming answer is, "right here.")
Not all contributors to the journals responded favorably to the CAM theme,
and I suspect that at least several would vigorously resist the suggestion that
they were even part of such a community. However, as Charland illustrates,
neither the meaning nor the membership of communities interpellated by discourse are stable because their boundaries and membership shift over time
and across circumstances.[6] Questions of membership permeate the definitions
of CAM advanced in the *JAMA-Archives* theme issues. Implicitly, they ask:
Who belongs in biomedicine? Who does not?

In their editorial in the *JAMA* theme issue, Fontanarosa and Lundberg
argue that the abundance of articles both submitted to and selected for inclusion in theme issues indicates that research on CAM is already under the
purview of the medical profession. They quantify this abundance as a critical
mass, noting that *JAMA* alone received over two hundred submissions, with
"many more" received by the *Archives* journals ("Alternative Medicine" 1618).
Enthusiastically, they report that "The result, after our usual rigorous review
process, is publication of more than 80 articles . . . in our 10 scientific journals, including 18 randomized trials and systematic reviews, on more than 30
different topics, and from more than 16 different countries" (1618). Fontanarosa and Lundberg's emphasis in this statement on peer assessment—"our
usual rigorous review process"—merits special attention because it serves
normalizing effects, reshaping research on potentially contentious health interventions as somewhat ordinary: the process belongs to the biomedical
community ("*our* . . . process"), it is routinized (the "*usual* . . . process"), and
it is stringent ("*rigorous* review").

The editors go on to specify that *JAMA* alone published six randomized
controlled trials (RCTs) of six "diverse alternative medicine therapies," in addition to a broad selection of other articles that they enumerate and describe
over the course of their editorial. Tellingly, none of the other editorials in
the annual theme issues published five years on either side of the 1998 CAM
issues feature any such quantification, nor do they emphasize the review process. In contrast, then, Fontanarosa and Lundberg's emphasis on the quantity

and quality of what they deem to be reliable research on CAM signals a self-conscious effort to present the theme issues as making legitimate contributions to biomedical knowledge.

Most of the contributing authors have MD degrees and were at the time of publication employed at conventional biomedical institutions, such as universities and hospitals. Only eight articles have authors with formal CAM accreditation: contributors to three articles hold doctoral-level biomedical designations (MD or PhD) in addition to CAM accreditation, and coauthors of five are trained solely in CAM (including acupuncture, traditional Chinese medicine, and naturopathy). Many contributors have dedicated their careers to studying CAM (e.g., Cardini and Weixin), while others are regular contributors to *JAMA* and the *Archives* on topics not primarily related to CAM (e.g., Delbanco). It is difficult to tell whether the small proportion of articles by authors with CAM credentials is a factor of submission or of editorial selection; in either case, the overwhelming presence of MDs and comparatively few CAM-trained researchers may have been a factor in the editors' assertions that the research reported in the theme issues is biomedically valid.[7]

Several contributors to the theme issues are prominent CAM researchers that have published widely in biomedical and CAM journals, with several publications each in the *JAMA-Archives* theme issues. Two of these researchers are important figures in this book. Physician-researcher David Eisenberg, the lead author of one article and coauthor of three others, has been at the forefront of research on CAM since the late 1970s, leading both the landmark 1993 survey in the *New England Journal of Medicine* of CAM use and expenditure and the 1998 follow-up survey in the *JAMA* theme issue. When the theme issues were published, Eisenberg was director of the Center for Alternative Medicine Research and Education at Harvard Medical School. He has since continued his research on alternative medicine in various posts, including as founding director of the integrative medicine-focused Osher Research Center at Harvard and the founding chief of Harvard's Division for Research and Education in Complementary and Integrative Medical Therapies.

Eisenberg's longtime collaborator and Harvard colleague, Ted Kaptchuk, contributed two articles to the theme issues, one as lead author. Kaptchuk holds an advanced degree in traditional Chinese medicine and has published prolifically on CAM, primarily in prestigious biomedical journals such as *JAMA*, the *Lancet*, and the *British Medical Journal*. Kaptchuk's analyses of research design and placebo effects have helped prompt intensive study of the role of intervention effects (i.e., effects of the act of treatment itself) on patient outcomes. Kaptchuk is currently Professor of Medicine and Director of

the Harvard-wide Program in Placebo Studies and the Therapeutic Encounter (known as PiPS), housed at Boston's Beth Israel Deaconess Medical Center. Both Kaptchuk and Eisenberg have maintained public visibility since the
1970s as boundary-straddling scholars in addition to their faculty appointments and active research programs, appearing in both print and television
as representatives of the "new science" of alternative medicine.[8]

Although the theme issues of *JAMA* and the *Archives* hail a biomedical
community that considers research on CAM as simply a matter of course,
many within the medical profession expressed concern about the potential
implications of such an expanded purview. For example, in a letter to the editor of *Archives of Pediatrics & Adolescent Medicine* in June 1998, five months
before the theme issues were published, physician Demetrios Theodoropoulos
expressed his "surprise" that the American Medical Association (AMA) journals would even entertain CAM as a special theme. He objected that publishing the theme issues will "unintentionally legitimize alternative medicine in a
journal under the auspices of the American Medical Association. . . . The purpose of this presentation is not clear and its implications will be harmful to the
profession and our patients" ("Professional Identity" 606). Theodoropoulos's
criticism is grounded in concern about the potential effects of applying the
AMA's imprimatur to the subject of CAM, which would effectively authorize
the practices under study. He concludes that, "if there is no 'alternative law' or
'alternative engineering,' why should our profession allow the laxity of attitude
to recognize an 'alternative'?" (606). The subsequent exchange that his letter
sparked within the journal offers insight into what is at stake in the *JAMA-
Archives* theme issues as a set of community-defining texts: the integrity and
scope of medicine itself.

In a response appended to Theodoropoulos's letter, the editor of *Archives of
Pediatrics & Adolescent Medicine*, Catherine DeAngelis, dismissed Theodoropoulos's concern: "I prefer to have what is submitted reviewed by those of us
who follow the traditional 'rules and regulations' before making a judgment"
(606). DeAngelis implies that scientific reason alone will ultimately determine
the merit of the submissions received, and that any perceived incursion on
professional territory can be settled by objective means. In a letter published in
the theme issue several months later, physician Gerald Ente offered a different
perspective, instead accusing Theodoropoulos of professional parochialism.
He described Theodoropoulos as offering only "the typical narrow-minded,
'scientific' physician's answer to a real problem that I believe is driving patients
away from allopathic medicine into the waiting, open arms of alternative,
complementary, integrative, or holistic medicine" (1154). For Ente, professional

borders are maintained not simply through pure reason but also through careful and flexible professional judgment: "We need not accept as truth all we learn, but we must keep learning" (1154).

Theodoropoulos was unpersuaded by either of these critiques. In a response to Ente's letter, also published in the journal's theme issue, Theodoropoulos restated still more candidly his concerns about professional turf: "The question of alternative medicine . . . is based on attacks to the integrity of medicine, the relevance of science, and the effectiveness of modern clinical practice. These views may occasionally be voiced in the American Medical Association press, but they do not promote our profession" (Reply 1154). Viewing the rise in popularity of CAM directly in terms of its potential effects on his own profession, Theodoropoulos concludes that mere "acknowledgement of alternative forms of medicine would inflict enough damage to a profession of allopathic physicians to outweigh any benefits (if there are any in the first place)" (1154).

This exchange among Theodoropoulos, DeAngelis, and Ente illustrates the variety of perspectives that members of the medical community held (and often still hold) regarding the professional implications of biomedical research on complementary and alternative medicine. Theodoropoulos's suggestion that even broaching the subject of CAM in a biomedical journal could threaten the medical profession may, at first, seem the most limited of the three perspectives. However, Theodoropoulos offers perhaps the most shrewd appraisal of the potential implications of bringing CAM into the scope of biomedical research, if only because he explicitly recognizes the roles of competition and publication in professional boundary work. In their more even-handed analyses, DeAngelis and Ente do not express such blatantly protectionist motives, and yet both authors place considerable stock in the ability of scientific method to adjudicate on matters that depend, in the end, on more than measurable phenomena—they depend also on the communities that measure them.

As Theodoropoulos points out, the contest over the boundaries of what counts as legitimate health care is determined significantly by the discursive activities of professions, such as the publication of professional journals. Because the texts that professions produce and use come, in effect, to constitute the professions themselves, Theodoropoulos's concern is well placed: publishing a study on the effect of lunar phases on postsurgical outcomes in an AMA-sponsored journal (Smolle, Prause, and Kerl), for example, implies that the AMA considers lunar phases a valid area of study. It seems almost beside the point that the result of this study, published in the theme issue of *Archives of Dermatology*, was negative, or that the authors themselves dismissed the intervention as "hav[ing] no relationship to the real world" (1369). Fontanarosa and Lundberg's emphasis in their *JAMA* editorial on the numeric quantity of CAM-themed articles assembled across the AMA journals, a seeming embarrassment of riches, glosses over the jurisdictional dispute occurring within their pages. By calling forth a biomedical community that appears already to encompass CAM research, the editors take as given biomedicine's jurisdiction over CAM, whereas Theodoropoulos takes that jurisdiction as not yet established.

Peer Review as Professional Self-Regulation

One means of establishing and protecting professional jurisdiction is through editorial assessment and peer review. The central function of both forms of review is to certify new knowledge by admitting once-tentative claims into a profession's shared store of knowledge (Berkenkotter, "Power"; Berkenkotter and Huckin; Gross, "Persuasion"; Sullivan). Fontanarosa and Lundberg cite editorial and peer review in exactly these terms, as the main assurance that the material included in the coordinated CAM-themed issues meets standards agreed upon by the biomedical community.[9] However, review does more than certify new knowledge: it is, equally, a form of professional self-regulation. As Gross notes, "Submission of a paper to a scientific journal counts as a request, a regulative act whose successful completion depends on shared social norms: Communicative action is initiated and issues, eventually, in a decision to accept or reject" ("Persuasion" 195). Despite peer review's ostensible purpose to control the quality of scholarship allowed into a discursive-professional community, review can also be used to block out other scholarship, even that of high quality, to protect either a reviewer's own interests or what he or she perceives as the interest of the discipline. Peer review both depends on and gives structure to the activities of professional communities.

For the boundaries of biomedicine within the 1998 CAM-themed issues of *JAMA* and the *Archives*, peer review cuts both ways. As DeAngelis and Ente argue, testing the submissions against the medical profession's established standards can eliminate those submissions that do not conform, a process that appears to ensure the integrity of the articles eventually published in the journals. However, as Theodoropoulos suggests, submissions that do pass the test do so ostensibly with the profession's official endorsement—and so, by accepting any articles at all, peer review might actually compromise the integrity of the community that produced those standards. On the latter point, physician C. N. M. Renckens colorfully argued several years after the theme issues that even "impeccable trials" of CAM ought to be dismissed on grounds of the "incomprehensible absurdit[y]" of the interventions under study (531). He warns that the consequence of even considering trials of CAM will be that "one's mind stays so open that the brains fall out!" (531).

One of the regulative acts that peer review performs is determining how biomedical CAM research will unfold: peer reviewers select which articles get published and which do not. Although I was not able to gain insight into the peer review process for the theme issues specifically,[10] *JAMA*'s own record of scholarship on editorial selection and peer review is revealing. Since the 1990s, the journal has regularly published articles calling for critical examination of peer review in biomedical journals, including in four dedicated theme issues that were based on presentations from the *JAMA*-sponsored International Congress on Editorial Peer Review in Biomedical Publication, which occurs every four years.[11] Directly countering Fontanarosa and Lundberg's claim that peer review ensures the integrity of the research reported in the CAM-themed issues, the research in *JAMA* on peer review problematizes peer review as an intellectual and social practice that operates under "the consciousness of the authority of science and the gatekeeping that undergirds it" (Burnham 1328; see also Horrobin; Knoll; and Rennie).

Of particular relevance to our consideration of the CAM-themed issues of *JAMA* and the *Archives* is the critique advanced in numerous of the *JAMA* theme issues on peer review that current review practices are inherently conservative. Elizabeth Knoll argued in 1990, for example, that "The peer review system is supposed to help along scientific discoveries and arguments. Like any bureaucracy, however, it copes best with routine—peer review works best when nothing much is at stake" (1332). In that same issue of *JAMA*, David Horrobin added weight to Knoll's argument by citing eighteen specific circumstances in which, in his view, the peer review process had "delayed, emasculated, or totally prevented the publication and investigation of potentially important findings" in studies of unusual or innovative interventions (1441). If Knoll and Horrobin are correct in their assessment that biomedical peer review "works best when nothing much is at stake" (Knoll), then we might infer that the peer review of submissions for the *JAMA-Archives* theme issues on CAM—which put at stake the boundaries of biomedicine itself—may not have worked well at all.

The basis of my inference here, that peer review was likely more problematic for the *JAMA-Archives* theme issues on CAM than for more conventional biomedical research, is that one of the governing principles of peer review is that researchers and reviewers belong to the same or similar discourse communities. This is exactly the issue that Debra Journet found in her study of one physician–author's efforts to meet the needs and expectations of his divergent audience of neurologists and psychoanalysts for his research on psychosomatic medicine. In research on CAM, however, the distance between researchers and reviewers may be far greater than that between researchers and reviewers of conventional biomedical studies, as CAM studies reach across not only different topics or medical specialties but different models of health and health care. Across that distance, researchers and reviewers may not have fully "shared social norms" (Gross, "Persuasion" 195), and so the biomedical standards by which submissions are evaluated may not suit the CAM interventions under study.

For instance, a biomedically trained reviewer with no experience in CAM research or practice may not be familiar with the methodological complexity of randomized controlled trials of interventions such as acupuncture, and so he or she may not be fully equipped to judge the strengths and weaknesses of such a trial. That reviewer may therefore reject the study on the basis that its design does not fit with his or her own expectations regarding procedures such as blinding and standardization, although such procedures are difficult to implement in many biomedical trials as well. For research on CAM, then, peer review constitutes a "regulative act" (Gross) because reviewers determine which studies are admitted to the profession's store of knowledge about CAM and which are not. This store of knowledge, in turn, helps determine the boundary between mainstream biomedicine and the various CAM practices it investigates.

If we consider the *JAMA-Archives* theme issues on CAM as an assemblage of profession-defining texts that constitute the community they address, then the picture of CAM that emerges within them sets the terms of how biomedical research on CAM will unfold. In the competitive ecosystem of the health professions, the biomedical community, as the dominant profession, can potentially redefine what CAM is, and even overwrite the histories and theoretical foundations of its constituent practices.

Categorizing Complementary and Alternative Medicine

Numerous commentators have identified the label "complementary and alternative medicine," or CAM, as forming a "residual category," a category best explained not by the logic uniting what it contains but by the logic excluding it from other categories within a classification system. For example, medical sociologist Paul Root Wolpe describes CAM as "defined not by its internal coherence but by its exclusion from other categories of medicine"

(165). Similarly, health policy expert Mary Ruggie argues that, primarily, "alternative medicine is understood in the negative—as something that is not medicine" (41). Compare this negative definition of CAM with the overarching logic of categorization within biomedicine, generally, articulated here by nursing scholar Annemarie Jutel: "There needs to be a reasonable rationale for placing similar objects together, ensuring that there is enough resemblance among members of the category for them to be associated" (15). Within biomedicine, items categorized together must fit meaningfully enough with one another to mobilize action. For example, medical specialties must hold together sufficiently as categories to organize medical research and training, whereas disease classifications must be robust enough to enable patient diagnosis and care (and insurance reimbursement). For the category of "CAM," however, the only rationale for placing together the health practices united under the category is their exclusion from biomedicine.

Examining CAM as a residual category in the *JAMA-Archives* theme issues allows us to understand how the various definitions that the journals give of CAM effect persuasion in the negotiation of biomedical boundaries. As Geoffrey Bowker and Susan Leigh Star observe about systems of classification, "Each standard and each category valorizes some point of view and silences another" (5). Defining CAM not by what it is but by what it is *not* is inherently political because it assumes the primacy of the biomedical model vis-à-vis other models of health and health care. The ways that the *JAMA-Archives* theme issues define CAM ultimately enhance and expand biomedical jurisdiction over matters of health and illness.

CAM's designation as residual, an umbrella for otherwise-unclassifiable practices, can be traced back at least to the Office of Alternative Medicine's (OAM) formal 1995 definition of CAM as "a broad domain of healing resources that encompasses all health systems, modalities, and practices and their accompanying theories and beliefs, other than those intrinsic to the politically dominant health system. . . . CAM includes all such practices and ideas self-defined by their users as preventing or treating illness or promoting health and well-being" (qtd. in Committee 19). This definition has been adopted widely in both the scholarly and popular press, often uncritically, even by those who advocate the various practices it encompasses. Though used increasingly in conjunction with "integrative medicine" since the *JAMA-Archives* theme issues were first published, the phrase "complementary and alternative medicine" continues to have significant traction despite its residual nature. Indeed, the compliance of supporters of individual CAM practices in using the CAM designation is itself good evidence of biomedicine's ability to set the terms under which the boundary debate unfolds.[12] As a residual category, "CAM" is powerful because its repeated and widespread use has naturalized its standing as a sociorhetorical construct.

In the *JAMA-Archives* theme issues, there is no consensus view of CAM, other than its ostensible opposition to biomedicine: some authors draw the boundary between biomedicine and CAM more restrictively than others. The articles cover a wide range of health interventions, from those with some credibility in biomedicine (such as acupuncture) to those on the extreme end of the alternative fringe (such as the effects of lunar phases on health), but nearly all of the articles contend that CAM threatens biomedicine's stability. The act of lumping such a disparate range of health practices together conceals whatever historical and philosophical coherence the practices might independently have, while at the same time accentuating, in contrast, biomedicine's own apparent coherence. Star and Bowker refer to concealing processes of this sort as the "double silencing" of residual categories, which involves "first putting [the thing classified] into a 'garbage' category . . . and then constructing the category in such a way that no historical or social information can escape from it" (274). Double-silenced as health practices with historical-professional narratives of their own (some of which span hundreds or thousands of years), the individual modalities that comprise CAM are effectively remade in the *JAMA-Archives* theme issues in biomedicine's own terms, all subsumed under the category "CAM."

CAM is defined most prominently in the theme issues as comprising "interventions not taught widely in medical schools nor generally available in US hospitals" (Eisenberg et al. "Trends" 1569). This definition, from Eisenberg and colleagues' lead article in *JAMA*, is cited across the journals but its meaning is never stable, not even within the Eisenberg et al. study itself. There, "CAM" refers ambiguously to a wide range of interventions, from those delivered by regulated professions with academic accreditation (e.g., chiropractic, massage therapy, traditional Chinese medicine) to those performed at home by individuals with little or no training (e.g., relaxation, self-help, prayer). This floating definition leaves many contributors to the theme issues unsure of what exactly counts as alternative medicine. Included among studies of acupuncture and herbal medicines, for example, are studies of yoga (Garfinkel et al.), spirituality (Thomsen), off-label use of dermatologic therapies (Li et al.), lanolin and breast shells for breastfeeding women (Brent et al.), and physician referral to clergy (Daaleman and Frey). Neither the authors of the off-label use study nor those of the breast shell study question their designation of those interventions as "alternative," even though both are common interventions in biomedicine.[13] The authors of the final study, Daaleman and Frey, admit to being unsure if physician referral to clergy counts as CAM, leaving the question open to readers.

While numerous of the journals under the AMA banner feature a wide range of alternative health practices in their theme issues (e.g., *JAMA*, *Archives of Dermatology*, *Archives of Internal Medicine*), others report on only a limited range. For example, the sole article on CAM in *Archives of Otolaryngology— Head & Neck Surgery*, an editorial, explains that only a "paradigm shift" will create space for CAM in the field of otolaryngology (Krouse 1200). In *Archives of General Psychiatry*, only two summary articles on CAM are included, under the heading "News and Views" (Ernst, Rand, and Stevinson; Wong, Smith, and Boon), while *Archives of Ophthalmology* does not broach the topic of CAM at all, not even in its regular news column, "In Other AMA Journals." In *Archives of Surgery*, aside from one systematic review of a homeopathic remedy (Ernst and Pittler), "alternative" takes on the very specific meaning of using new or different surgical techniques, such as minimally invasive surgery. One pair of authors within that journal urges surgeons to avoid the "alternative" label altogether because of its association with CAM: "Alternative medicine, as it applies to trauma management, might be safely considered an oxymoron" (Britt and Cole 1177).

We might entertain several explanations of the limited coverage of CAM in these specialty journals. CAM interventions may simply be more applicable to some areas of medicine than to others. This interpretation is compatible with the main conditions for which individuals seek CAM, including chronic, functional conditions such as back, muscle, or joint pain, headache, and digestive problems. Such conditions are more likely to be treated in primary care settings, and so the higher emphasis on CAM in journals such as *Archives of Family Medicine* than in specialty journals makes sense. An alternate, possibly compatible explanation is that some specialties, particularly more prestigious ones such as surgery, may be more fortified professionally against boundary incursion than others. Acupuncture, chiropractic, and massage therapy are all widely promoted as nonsurgical alternatives for musculoskeletal disorders, so it is curious not to find in *Archives of Surgery* some discussion of their safety and efficacy as compared to surgery. Whatever the explanation for the comparatively lower coverage of CAM in these specialty journals than in the other journals of the *JAMA-Archives* theme issues, this lower coverage indicates that some areas of biomedicine are less available to, or better guarded against, the encroachment of CAM than others. The model of CAM that emerges in the *JAMA-Archives* theme issues, then, is somewhat restricted, possibly sensitive to internal biomedical hierarchies.

Definitions of CAM within the theme issues, while variable, generally pivot on the demarcation of boundaries between science and nonscience. Demarcation, in Gieryn's view, aims to "identify unique and essential characteristics of science that distinguish it from other kinds of intellectual activities" ("Boundary-Work" 781). Sociologist Robert Evans similarly describes demarcation as the search for "what, if anything, makes science special" within the larger culture (3). Within the *JAMA-Archives*, questions about the demarcation between biomedicine and CAM are generally implicit, as in the exchange I discussed above between Theodoropoulos, DeAngelis, and Ente. Theodoropoulos premised his concern about the theme issues' effects on the medical profession on the idea that biomedicine and CAM occupy separate domains—they are scientific and nonscientific, respectively. Tom Delbanco assumed a similar position in *JAMA*, likening research on CAM to the "scientific study of astrology" (1561). For Delbanco, science is simply not an appropriate arena for evaluating CAM, and so clinical trials of practices such as homeopathy constitute a category error: the trial of art or magic by the methods of science. DeAngelis and Ente take the opposite tack in their exchange with Theodoropoulos, claiming that the methods of science are the only means through which we can discern which practices are supportable by evidence and which are not.

For those authors who do explicitly discuss matters of demarcation in the *JAMA-Archives* theme issues, the relationship between biomedical boundaries and distinctions between science and nonscience is variable. Some authors vigorously (and often humorously) decry alternative medicine in the name of boundary work as unscientific. In *Archives of Dermatology*, for example, Rudolf Happle contends that CAM "represents a collective aberration of mind" (1455). He argues that medical professionals must establish an "epistemological demarcation" between what he calls "rational" (mainstream) and "irrational" (alternative) medicine (1455). The litmus test for identifying "rational" health practices, according to Happle, is whether or not they can be falsified—a principle from Karl Popper that holds that that a theory can only count as scientific if it can be subjected to empirical testing and be either proven or disproven; anything that cannot be empirically proven or disproven (such as a theory of God) would then be categorized as nonscientific.[14] As Evans points out, the falsification principle is a problematic demarcation criterion because falsification is itself a mobile concept, open to negotiation and not solely driven by data (6). Happle is uncompromising in the boundaries he wishes to draw, however. He warns those who would defend alternative medicine: "if you who are reading this article do not know what rational thinking means, you are beyond help" (1457).

While Happle dismisses CAM on the grounds that it is inherently unscientific, and so in his view is inadmissible to biomedicine, other contributors to the *JAMA-Archives* theme issues take seriously the challenge to understand how CAM fits vis-à-vis biomedicine. For example, in *Archives of Internal Medicine*, Goodwin and Tangum couch their discussion of nutritional supplements within an account of professional dynamics that resonates with Andrew Abbott's model of professions as a competitive ecosystem. They maintain that proponents of micronutrient supplements of the twentieth century had been dismissed on the same grounds for which Galileo faced resistance in the seventeenth century: because they "did not respect professional boundaries" (2187). Even if a given intervention is advanced by "outsiders" selling directly to the public (2187), they argue, medical researchers and practitioners must undertake good-faith attempts to determine if those interventions are safe and effective. Systemic biases against vitamin research on such grounds have, in their view, consequently produced bodies of data that are founded on incomplete or faulty evidence.

Lest readers assume that Goodwin and Tangum are "apologists for megavitamins," the authors clarify that their interest lies only in what the "vitamin controversy" can tell us about how cultural forces can affect medical practice (2187). Citing philosophers of science Feyerabend and Kuhn, as well as Michel Foucault, they emphasize the important opportunities that biomedical research on CAM affords for understanding how social context "influences everything we do as physicians—which diseases we recognize and which we ignore, which treatments we use, and which we reject. The more we learn about why we do what we do, the more likely we are to avoid errors in the future" (2190). While Happle invokes a firm division between biomedicine (as "rational") and CAM (as "irrational"), Goodwin and Tangum instead depict that boundary as permeable and subject to social and cultural forces. Included among those forces are concerns over professional jurisdiction.

Sugarman and Burk's article on health policy and CAM in the *JAMA* theme issue moves the arena of debate about CAM from questions of demarcation to questions of practice. They argue that, although discussions of boundaries are useful for identifying practices that belong to distinct epistemic realms, the real work of medicine is treating patients. Distinctions between science and nonscience do not matter in the practice of medicine, they assert, since patients are not bound to the same epistemological allegiances as physicians. The problem, for Sugarman and Burk, therefore lies not in whether or not CAM counts as scientific but instead in the scarcity of research-derived evidence about CAM. Such evidence is necessary for physicians to effectively advise patients and yet, the authors argue, there is little political or professional will in biomedicine to investigate CAM interventions. They remind their readers that, in helping patients meet health-related goals, physicians have an ethical obligation to accept CAM's popularity and gain knowledge about it rather than dismiss it out of hand, especially since patients use CAM whether or not their physicians know or approve. Sugarman and Burk offer a timely reminder that boundary work affects more than the professions that engage in it: physicians' attitudes toward and knowledge about CAM directly affect their patients' care.

In considering the rhetorical demarcation of medical boundaries vis-à-vis CAM, Sugarman and Burk illustrate how lumping the many health interventions that do not fit under biomedicine into a single category of leftovers—CAM—makes those practices essentially "unknowable" on their own terms (Star and Bowker). The individual practices that comprise CAM are instead funneled into a broad category premised on its discontinuity with biomedicine, making it harder to see the continuity of their core values with biomedicine, such as promoting health, preventing illness, and alleviating suffering (1624). Of course, these shared values alone do not render practices such as acupuncture or chiropractic commensurable with biomedicine. However, as Sugarman and Burk argue, reflexive efforts to discount CAM solely on the basis of its scientific standing miss the opportunity to learn more about how best to meet patients' needs.

As a conceptual category, "CAM" therefore risks galvanizing those who wish to dismiss the practices it describes simply on definitional grounds, on the argument that "if it's not biomedicine, then it must not be legitimate." Consider, for instance, the various definitions of CAM offered in the *JAMA-Archives* theme issues: taken individually, many articles discuss complementary and alternative medicine thoughtfully and with nuance, and some even move beyond simple binary distinctions between biomedicine and not-biomedicine. However, when we take those definitions together, CAM is so many different things at once that it is, in essence, nothing in particular—it is, in other words, a residual category.

This residual definition of CAM constitutes the first movement of what Star and Bowker call the "double silencing" of residual categories, compiling phenomena that do not fit within a classification system into a category of leftovers. From the perspective of persuasion, this negative classification undermines the residual category of "CAM" itself: uniting practices that are otherwise unrelated renders the category itself incoherent. The incoherence of that category, in turn, makes it all the easier to dismiss individual modalities contained within the category as similarly incoherent. For example, lumping chiropractic and massage therapy, both licensed and regulated health professions founded on largely biomechanical understandings of the body, into the same category as faith-based or mystical interventions (e.g., prayer and lunar phases) may affect the extent to which biomedical personnel will entertain those practices as plausible. Therefore, by defining the various interventions that comprise CAM in residual terms as a collective, "CAM," the theme issues advance a metalevel claim that figures biomedicine as the benchmark that will set the terms of what CAM is and what it will be.

CAM à la Carte

In this final section, I examine the second movement of double-silencing within the *JAMA-Archives* theme issues as a discursive artifact of the medical profession, in which CAM, as a residual category, is "then construct[ed] . . . in such a way that no historical or social information can escape from it" (Star and Bowker 274). As Star and Bowker argue, once a residual category is formed, that category obscures the individual, idiosyncratic characteristics of the phenomena it contains, redefining those phenomena instead in terms of the category into which they have been absorbed. In the *JAMA-Archives* theme issues, CAM practices are redefined in terms more congruent with biomedical theory and practice. This filtering of nonbiomedical health practices through a biomedical terminology is only to be expected, since scholarly journals must speak the language of their readers. However, to understand how the notion of evidence determines the boundaries of biomedicine, generally, we need know whether, and to what extent, the evidence produced in peer-reviewed journals for a given CAM intervention is representative of, and applicable to, that intervention in practice.

The CAM interventions under evaluation in the *JAMA-Archives* theme issues often bear little resemblance to how they are practiced in their native contexts of use. When the articles offer historical genealogies of the CAM practices they investigate, those histories allow surprisingly little "historical or social information" about the practices to "escape from" the biomedical discourse into which they have been imported, to draw on Star and Bowker's formulation. By compiling together all practices not explainable under the biomedical model, biomedicine itself appears more stable and coherent in relief, even though it does not itself encompass a fully fixed set of medical values or practices (see Stein). As a residual category, then, CAM not only obscures the histories of the practices it comprises—it also obscures biomedicine's own unstable past.

Some articles within *JAMA* and the *Archives* do provide reflective accounts of individual CAM practices within their historical contexts. The most comprehensive of these articles is Oumeish Youssef Oumeish's review in *Archives of Dermatology* of the complex social, cultural, and scientific histories of healing traditions across the globe and across centuries. His fourteen-page article offers encyclopedic summaries of the central tenets and applications of a staggering array of CAM interventions ranging from chiropractic, crystal therapy, and cupping to leech therapy and naturopathy. This is Oumeish's entry for homeopathy, perhaps the most reviled of the dominant CAM practices within biomedicine (see Negele), which is premised on a mechanism of action that is fully incompatible with scientific principles:

> Homeopathy is a system of medicine based on the theory of "like cures like."
> For example, a poison that causes symptoms of illness in a healthy person
> can treat the same symptoms in a diluted form. Substances are diluted several
> times to make a remedy that is safe to use, yet homeopaths believe sufficient
> likeness remains between the remedy and the illness to stimulate the body's
> self-healing abilities. It is based on the pharmacological "law of similars" that
> was invented in 1796 by Samuel Hahnemann, a German physician. The word
> derives from the Greek "homoios" and "pathos," meaning to suffer. Another
> example is rubbing chilblains with snow. Homeopathy also encourages people
> to reject strong medications. (1384)

Oumeish makes his own position on homeopathy clear—it is founded on an "invented" theory that "homeopaths *believe*" restores patients to health—but his careful description of the modality's core philosophy and principles of practice provides a full-bodied account of what patients believe about homeopathy and why they engage in it. The richness of Oumeish's description of each of the practices he describes (not to mention his article's extravagant length within a medical journal, at fourteen pages) serves as a stark point of contrast to the overwhelming majority of articles within the theme issues.

In contrast to Oumeish, most authors in *JAMA* and the *Archives* limit their discussion of different CAM practices to those practices' contact with biomedicine. By minimizing the philosophical, practical, and professional independence of the CAM intervention under study, the medical profession can more easily claim jurisdiction over the empirical investigation of that intervention. Most of the clinical trial reports within the theme issues, for instance, treat the interventions under study as a kind of medicine à la carte, in which certain CAM principles can be adopted, piecemeal, into biomedicine. Under the constraining genre of the clinical trial report, the IMRaD structure (introduction, methods, results, and discussion), there appears to be no space for anything but the straight facts, and so the articles' lack of attention to CAM as a social or historical phenomenon is fully conventional and not itself noteworthy. However, the articles' inattention to the complex specifics of each CAM intervention under study does significantly affect how the studies are designed, which may in turn affect the relevance of their results to practice: if trials of CAM do not reproduce the interventions as they are enacted in real-life settings, the results they produce may not hold clinical significance.

For example, Shlay et al.'s trial of acupuncture for AIDS-related pain control in *JAMA* does not describe or evaluate the practice as an integral component of a comprehensive, autonomous health system, traditional Chinese medicine (TCM). Instead, the researchers adopt a research protocol fundamentally at odds with the TCM model, using a standardized acupuncture procedure that they admit "differs from the practice of most acupuncturists, who treat patients with individualized regimens" (1594). The ease with which the authors dismiss this shortcoming, especially given their study's negative finding, indicates their reluctance to consider acupuncture as part of a complete, independent model of health care. Whether that reluctance is conscious or unconscious is beside the point—the fact remains that acupuncture is reduced in this article to the mere insertion of needles into flesh. Although acupuncture has long been a subject of interest in American health care (see, e.g., the *American Journal of Chinese Medicine*, founded in 1973), in Shlay et al.'s article, it is as if acupuncture has no history of its own.

Likewise, Garfinkel et al.'s trial of yoga for the treatment of carpal tunnel syndrome, also in *JAMA*, does not account for yoga's cultural history as a constituent element of Ayurvedic medicine. Like TCM, Ayurveda is a complete, ancient philosophy of health encompassing prevention, diagnosis, and treatment (although not necessarily in those terms). The authors attribute their study's partially positive findings to biomechanical improvements, such as relieved compression, better joint posture, and improved blood flow, whereas, in Ayurveda, such improvement would instead be attributed to shifts in elements such as heat and wind. Certainly, we cannot chastise biomedical researchers for not citing heat and wind as mechanisms of action in their studies. Even still, the omission of these basic principles of Ayurveda as matters that may at least be relevant to implementing the yoga techniques in biomedical practice is telling.

These two articles, on acupuncture and yoga respectively, are typical of the research articles in the *JAMA-Archives* theme issues on complementary and alternative medicine: they offer brief anecdotes, historical trivia, or statistical information on usage or spending regarding the interventions under study and then evaluate those interventions as though they exist independently of the philosophies of health from which they are derived. With CAM constructed primarily as a residual category, these studies thus minimize their associations with CAM, allowing researchers to proceed with potentially boundary-threatening work without compromising the authority of biomedicine or their standing within it. In this view, the absence of history regarding the individual practices that comprise CAM works persuasively because it allows researchers to study practices such as TCM not as unique, autonomous, philosophically grounded practices but as a disparate set of discrete techniques, such as acupuncture, that can simply be absorbed by biomedicine (or not).

Of course, unlike TCM and Ayurveda, not all CAM practices are autonomous or philosophically grounded, and this is one of the most problematic aspects of CAM as a descriptive category. As I have argued in this chapter, CAM aggregates into a single category a jumble of health interventions that are not necessarily of the same conceptual order: some are self-administered and unstructured (e.g., prayer), while others are fully professionalized with formal education and licensing (e.g., chiropractic); some consist of stand-alone treatments (e.g., megavitamins), while others are comprehensive health systems (e.g., Ayurveda); and some have philosophies of practice that are essentially compatible with biomedicine (e.g., massage therapy), while others stand in opposition (e.g., TCM)—and still others operate parasitically on the biomedical model (e.g., live blood analysis).

Before concluding this chapter, I want to restrict my own definition of CAM, which will guide my discussion over the remainder of this book. Referring to such an unwieldy range of interventions included under the category of CAM would require so much explanatory apparatus along the way that my analysis of biomedical boundary work would become unmanageable, particularly because I do not want to elide categories myself. And so, in the chapters to come, I focus on acupuncture, chiropractic, and dietary supplements (e.g., herbal remedies and megavitamins), which, for convenience, I also refer to collectively as "CAM." These interventions are united by three factors, although they remain otherwise distinct: they are the practices most accessed by patients, they are the most researched, and they have the highest levels of physician support and referral.[15] However, as I refer to "CAM" as these three practices, I want also to retain a penumbral reference to the other interventions that are cast in the theme issues as *alternative* to biomedicine.

The interventions within my restricted definition have posed the most formidable challenge to biomedicine as a profession but, as use of practices such as energy therapies and homeopathy rises further, and as research agendas follow suit, those less-studied interventions may follow a similar trajectory.

*

Writing on the rhetoric of the scientific article, rhetoric scholar Herbert Simons observes that "researchers are not free agents" (152). Rather, "they are impelled and constrained by the conventions of their disciplines, by the norms and counternorms of their professions, and by political and economic pressures coming from the larger society" (152). Viewed in this light, the fact that the authors of the clinical trial reports on acupuncture and yoga that I discuss above do not reflect substantively on the philosophical implications of their research may not be surprising, given the generic constraints within which they write. However, the genre of the scientific article does more than marshal its authors' words into a recognizable format: it abstracts the interventions under study from their usual contexts of delivery and remakes them in biomedical terms. The reconstruction of complementary and alternative medicine in biomedicine's own image makes scientific research on CAM possible, but what is often overlooked in debates about the legitimacy of unconventional health practices and practitioners is that this reconstruction also serves a central argumentative function. As I show in the next chapter, the evidence produced in the name of evidence-based medicine can tilt the course of arguments to defend or expand professional boundaries.

Although many commentators within the *JAMA-Archives* theme issues contend that the debate about CAM can be settled with enough evidence, they often underestimate how dependent that evidence is on the communities that produce it. Given biomedicine's greater rhetorical resources as the dominant model in the health care ecosystem, the evidence that biomedicine produces can shore up its authority and expand its jurisdiction to health practices formerly beyond its scope. As a rhetorical "moment" in the history of medicine as a profession, then, the publication of the *JAMA-Archives* theme issues on CAM offers insight into the ability of discourse to constitute professional communities and to categorize certain fields of theory, research, and practice as either within or beyond the bounds of those communities. In his editorial in the theme issue of *JAMA*, Wayne Jonas, then the head of the Office of Alternative Medicine (which was about to become the National Center for Complementary and Alternative Medicine), reflects on this process:

Historically, orthodox medicine fights [CAM] practices vigorously by de-nouncing and attacking them, restricting access to them, labeling them as an-tiscientific and quackery, and imposing penalties for practicing them. When these therapies persist and even rise in popularity despite this, mainstream medicine then turns more friendly, examining them, identifying similarities they have with the orthodox, and incorporating or "integrating" them into the routine practice of medicine. (1616)

The late historian of medicine Roy Porter is more direct, if cynical, in his account of competition in the medical marketplace in the seventeenth and eighteenth centuries, as he sums up one of this book's central claims: "quack-ery never prospers, for if and when it does, it becomes termed medicine in-stead" (207).

3

Scientific Methods at the Edge of Biomedicine

As evidence-based medicine (EBM) rose to prominence over the final decade of the twentieth century and the first decade of the twenty-first, the medical profession increasingly linked its self-identity and scientific and cultural authority to its grounding of clinical decision-making in evidence derived from randomized controlled trials (RCTs), biomedicine's defining, gold-standard research method. The rhetoric of EBM has become an epideictic rhetoric in contemporary Western culture, a rhetoric of praise and blame in which *evidence* is taken as a good in itself and the central premise seems simply to be "the more, the better." However, it is a slippery rhetoric, too, because, while evidence is lavishly praised in the abstract, certain kinds of evidence are more praiseworthy in certain contexts than are others. In deliberation about health practices that sit on or beyond the boundaries of biomedicine, the evidence produced by RCTs can be construed, invoked, and employed strategically to expand or contract the limits of what counts as safe, effective health care and what does not.[1] Biomedicine is therefore bounded, in part, by how researchers design and interpret clinical studies.

At the core of the November 1998 theme issues of the *Journal of the American Medical Association* and the *Archives* specialty journals lies a conflict about how research on complementary and alternative medicine (CAM) ought to be conducted, interpreted, and incorporated into biomedical practice. Most CAM interventions are not easily randomized, generalized across populations, controlled, or blinded, and so they are difficult to test within the framework of the RCT. This difficulty of testing stems from CAM practices' general incommensurability with biomedicine, both in theory and practice. The methodological challenges that biomedical research on CAM poses are a central issue around which the contributors to the *JAMA-Archives* theme issues align their texts to position CAM within or beyond scientific borders, depending on their own stance toward CAM and the practices it comprises.

In this chapter, I examine the problem of method in scientific research on CAM as a fundamentally rhetorical problem that is situated within a boundary drama and deeply rooted in the discursive practices of science and medicine. Not even mainstream biomedical research is conducted entirely through RCTs—observational and qualitative studies also fill the pages of medical journals. As philosopher of science Kirstin Borgerson notes, most biomedical interventions in North America have not been tested in stringent RCTs and so "Research into alternative medicine is required to meet the highest standards even though many currently accepted medical practices have not met (and may never meet) those same standards" (506n1). Even among those authors in the *JAMA-Archives* theme issues who are friendly to CAM (e.g., Fontanarosa and Lundberg; Margolin, Avants, and Kleber), the consensus on CAM research is that practices such as acupuncture and chiropractic must be held up to a higher standard of evidence—medical ethics and policy specialist Haavi Morreim deems it a double standard (228)—than biomedicine.

In debates about CAM, methods of evidence production often serve as a proxy for establishing the "reasonableness" of claims regarding individual CAM interventions. In Lawrence J. Prelli's rhetorical framework for understanding scientific discourse, claims deemed within science to be "reasonable" are those that "possess empirical accuracy, consistency, quantitative precision, or explanatory power," whereas "unreasonable" claims are those that are "empirically inaccurate, inconsistent, quantitatively imprecise, or lacking explanatory strength" ("Rhetorical Logic" 317–18). Because the practices that comprise CAM generally fall beyond the boundaries of everyday scientific practice, they hold no claims of their own to reasonableness within the scientific community. Such claims are instead established in debates about CAM by drawing on the notion of method as a rhetorical topos—a "perspective from which to argue" (Prelli, *Rhetoric* 77–78)—that invokes the randomized controlled trial as a surrogate metric of reasonableness. The extent to which a CAM practice can successfully be tested in an RCT serves as a marker of whether or not that practice is "reasonable" within biomedicine.

According to Aristotle, a rhetorical topos (plural: topoi) is an inventional framework for generating arguments either in general contexts, with the "common topoi" (possible and impossible, past fact, future fact, and size), or in specific circumstances, with the "special topoi" (e.g., consequences, definition, more or less). In rhetoric of science, prevalent special topoi include consistency and disinterestedness (Prelli, *Rhetoric*), as well as "scales," the weighing of pros and cons or risks and benefits (Scott, *Risky* 61). In this chapter, I show that commentators on all sides of debates about complementary and alternative medicine draw on the argumentative resources of the method topos to establish claims about what constitutes valid biomedical research. By "method," I am referring, abstractly, to a way of doing or a procedure for acting. In the *JAMA-Archives* theme issues, arguments generated by this topos generally invoke method in the specific sense of doing research in randomized controlled trials, which position the RCT as the only appropriate way of producing valid evidence about CAM.

I examine the topos of method through close analysis of two randomized controlled trials of acupuncture published in the *JAMA* theme issue and through five discourse-based interviews that I conducted with expert readers about those studies' methods and results. (I describe the two articles below and my interview methods in the introduction.) The first section begins by contextualizing the method topos within the overlapping orbits of evidence-based medicine, clinical trial design, and CAM. The second section examines how the genre of the experimental article is itself mobilized in biomedical research on CAM to determine which forms of medicine come to count as evidence-based. Reports of clinical trials are modeled on the conventional publication genre of the sciences, which follows the IMRaD format (introduction, methods, results, and discussion); because this format conditions our beliefs about how science and medicine are conducted (and, importantly, *not* conducted), it can illuminate how method can be invoked rhetorically. The third section takes up the specifics of arguments from method in biomedical research on CAM, while the fourth section isolates the concept of *efficacy*, whether or not a health intervention "works," as a central organizing principle of that research. Although the determination of efficacy appears to follow inevitably from the randomized controlled trial as a research method, this final section suggests that the process of determination itself is loaded with rhetorical power that can have significant implications for biomedical boundary work.

Of the thirteen clinical trial reports in the *JAMA-Archives* theme issues, I focus specifically on two trials of acupuncture. Biomedical researchers and physicians regard acupuncture as one of the most effective CAM interventions (Astin et al.) and most supported by compelling data (Hsu and Diehl; Shang). Its credibility within mainstream medicine has been bolstered, especially, by emergent data on its effectiveness for pain control ("NIH Consensus"). Credibility within biomedicine is an important asset for a CAM practice in the context of boundary work because, without that credibility, even the most rigorously designed studies might easily be dismissed on that ground alone. Sociologist Nina Degele has found this to be the case with research on homeopathy and parapsychology, for example, practices that are so implausible, scientifically, that even the most stringent trial design could not overcome the skepticism of most mainstream scientific readers (111).

Acupuncture has been well-studied within biomedicine over the past thirty years but it continues to present considerable methodological challenges because the philosophy underlying its mechanism of action, stimulating the flow of *qi* ("chi," or energy) along meridians accessible by acupuncture needles, is incommensurable with biomedical theory. Unlike trials of herbal supplements, which are comparatively more amenable to the randomized controlled trial format, trials of acupuncture provide a window into the workaday elements of biomedical boundary work because their methodological challenges allow us to track the accommodations that researchers must make to fit their studies within accepted research standards.

Cardini and Weixin's trial, published in the *JAMA* theme issue, investigated the technique of moxibustion for the reversal of breech pregnancies in Chinese maternity clinics. Moxibustion, the practice of burning cigar-shaped *moxa* rolls of *Artemisia vulgaris* (mugwort) on acupuncture points to stimulate the flow of *qi*, has long been the standard treatment in traditional Chinese medicine (TCM) for breech presentation. Participants in the study's intervention arm were treated by their partners every day for two weeks between 33 and 35 weeks' gestation by burning a *moxa* roll on the outside of the right pinkie toenail, whereas participants in the control group received routine maternity care. The study's primary outcome measures were for cephalic (head-first) presentation at thirty-five weeks' gestation, checked by ultrasound, and at birth. The study's result was positive, leading the authors to conclude that moxibustion was effective for reversing breech presentation.

Shlay et al.'s study, also published in the *JAMA* theme issue, compared acupuncture with both a placebo intervention and the current pharmaceutical standard of care, amitriptyline, for the treatment of HIV-related peripheral neuropathy (pain, sensitivity, and numbness in the extremities). This multicenter study, conducted at HIV primary care centers in ten US cities, featured a modified factorial design with multiple treatment arms that compared acupuncture to placebo (or "sham") acupuncture, amitriptyline to a placebo pill, and all combinations of these interventions to each other. Outcomes were assessed through subjective patient reports in pain diaries and pain scores, which showed that neither acupuncture nor amitriptyline were more effective than placebos for HIV-related pain in the extremities.[2]

Biomedical research on CAM, I want ultimately to show in this chapter, precipitates what Bertolt Brecht called (in a context unrelated to either medicine or rhetoric) the *Verfremdungseffekt*—the "estrangement effect": it makes the normally tacit procedures of medical research "strange" and, as a consequence, more readily open to inquiry.[3] Studies of CAM bring the biomedical research apparatus into question, particularly because, while there is clearly knowledge to be gained from studying CAM, there is no established method of proceeding. Observing researchers as they attempt to perform effective and rigorous research on CAM, most notably how they design their studies and interpret their results, can open up the epistemic machinery of medicine as a whole. As Morreim explains, "Any attempt to throw out or discredit CAM on grounds of scientific inadequacy is sure to toss out large portions of conventional medicine alongside. To 'hold' both to 'the same' standards appears to bode far worse for medicine than for CAM" (228).

By tracing how even biomedicine often fails the standards of research set by critics of CAM, we can learn more about the rhetorical workings of evidence derived from randomized controlled trials, the centerpiece of evidence-based medicine. One of my overarching aims in this chapter, then, is to show that arguments about method in debates about complementary and alternative medicine can be read, metonymically, as expressions of more general anxieties in biomedicine about knowledge and evidence, community values, and professional boundaries.

I ought to note at the outset that although rhetoric, as a theoretical and pedagogical practice, is not about unmasking per se, this chapter does a little unmasking to illuminate some of the disconnections between how medical researchers and practitioners (and policymakers, the media, and the public) think about the conduct and value of medical research, and how that research tends actually to unfold. I do not mean to suggest, however, that these disconnections between theory and practice are intentionally deceptive; indeed, the disconnections seem to be at least partly functional, making possible the everyday work of medicine. Instead, I want to show that the value system that attends the randomized controlled trial is part of the professional fabric of medicine itself. By illuminating disconnections between theory and practice in research, we can map some of the epistemological dimensions of rhetorical boundary work in biomedicine more generally.

Idealizing Evidence: Scientific Methods and CAM Research

The argument from method in the CAM-themed issues of *JAMA* and the *Archives* is founded on the entrenchment of the randomized controlled trial as the principal source of evidence in evidence-based medicine. Methodology has long functioned as a "rhetorical resource" in scientific boundary work

(Yeo 261), but the positioning of CAM within the paradigm of EBM further expands the argumentative scope of the method topos as it reaches across the diverse conceptual geographies of science, medicine, and alternative approaches to health. I explain in this section how CAM practices resist the format of the randomized controlled trial and track how researchers in the *JAMA-Archives* theme issues such as Cardini and Weixin and Shlay et al. design their trials to fit within accepted evidence-based standards.

An article in the *New York Times Magazine* from 2007 captures in miniature what this chapter argues is a deep ambivalence in the medical literature about methodology and evidence. In that article, journalist and science writer Gary Taubes asks, "Do we really know what makes us healthy?" Focusing on the case of hormone replacement therapy (HRT), Taubes critiques the evidence used to make public health recommendations, noting that today's recommendations often wind up as tomorrow's prohibitions.[4] Taubes cautions readers against putting too much stock in either observational or experimental studies, both of which he argues are more problematic than they first appear. Despite his round criticism of all forms of evidence production, however, Taubes ultimately favors an experimental approach. Marshaling the words of evidence-based medicine's father figure, David Sackett, Taubes frames the case of hormone replacement therapy, which was based on observational research, as an object-lesson in the "'disastrous inadequacy of lesser evidence.'" Even if trial data are problematic, Taubes urges readers "to remain skeptical until somebody spends the time and the money to do a randomized trial."

Taubes's argument that observational studies can only suggest correlations between health interventions and outcomes while RCTs can give more concrete answers is uncontroversial. What is significant about his article is the elasticity of his notion of evidence: Taubes is able to argue, in virtually the same breath, that we *cannot* trust the evidence from either kind of study but that we *can* trust RCT-derived evidence. It is as though he invokes, silently, the ubiquitous evidence hierarchies of the EBM literature, which rank the quality of evidence from RCTs and systematic reviews at the top and that derived from observational and other nonexperimental studies at the bottom (see table 2).[5] That is, the relative stability of RCT-derived evidence shifts over the course of Taubes's article: on its own terms, the RCT is given clear-eyed assessment, warts and all, but as the ranking methodology within the larger context of evidence production, it gains a kind of concrete authority. This shift is not surprising because, as philosopher of medicine Uffe Juul Jensen has noted of EBM, "what is accepted as evidence always depends on

TABLE 2. Sample evidence hierarchy

Hierarchy of evidence for medical research (in descending order of reliability)
Systematic review of several large randomized controlled trials
Single large randomized controlled trial
Systematic review of several small randomized controlled trials
Single small randomized controlled trial
Systematic review of several case-control or cohort studies
Single case-control or cohort study
Systematic review of several cross-sectional studies
Single cross-sectional study
Case series
Expert opinion (by individual authority with clinical experience or committee)

ontologies enacted in a particular context. Different ontologies will embody or imply different standards" (104). In rhetorical terms, different evidence is differently persuasive in different contexts.

The kinds of evidence considered admissible in biomedical debates about alternative medicine vary depending on where they are invoked and by whom. In mainstream medical journals, those writing on CAM frequently occupy an ambivalent position: attentive to diverse ways of understanding and assessing health in accordance with the rhetoric of CAM (valuing both quantitative and qualitative evidence, for example) but inattentive to that diversity when installing CAM within the discourse of biomedicine (relying solely on quantitative evidence).

This privileging of certain kinds of proof within research contexts is systemic, with researchers constrained by the genres of their own practice, particularly the genre of the clinical trial report. The tension between different standards of evidence stands in sharp relief when we read the clinical trials and systematic reviews of the theme issues against other genres published within the *JAMA-Archives* theme issues, such as editorials, historical essays, and letters. These latter articles advocate different criteria for what should as evidence for the efficacy of health interventions. Rhetoric scholar Judy Segal notes that "editorial writings supply good evidence that the 'neutral' nature of scientific texts is a matter neither of the basic inclinations of scientific authors nor the nature of their subject matter; the neutral style is a cultivated style which has become conventionalized in a particular forum for scientific writing: the scientific article" ("Strategies" 528). Segal shows that experimental articles, such as clinical trial reports, are not simply discursive records of objective procedures, although they appear to be. Rather, scientific articles are, as Burke would say, part of the "tribal idioms . . . *developed* by their use as instruments in the tribe's way of living" (*Language* 44; emphasis in original). Put another way, no less than editorial writings, experimental articles are, again using Burke's terms, the "dancing of an attitude" (*Philosophy* 9).

Editorial essays in medical journals are themselves constrained by generic conventions, but those conventions are comparatively less restrictive than those of clinical trial reports. Editorials permit greater candor, allowing scientific authors to reflect more openly on issues that affect their profession, in turn giving the reader a better sense of the authors' "basic inclinations" (Segal, "Strategies" 528), varied as those may be. In disputes about biomedicine's boundaries, analyzing research articles vis-à-vis editorials can destabilize long-held beliefs about the methods adopted in the service of evidence production. Destabilizing those beliefs in turn brings into focus the argument from method invoked in the CAM-themed issues of *JAMA* and the *Archives*.

In his lead editorial in *JAMA*, for example, Wayne Jonas, then-director of the National Institutes of Health's Office of Alternative Medicine, praises practitioners of CAM for helping to "address the confusion and suffering that accompany disease" (1616); he encourages biomedical doctors to emulate CAM practitioners in their attention to patients' experience of illness. Jonas's concern about biomedicine's reduced capacity for interpersonal care is repeated across the editorial articles in the *JAMA-Archives* theme issues. One set of authors argues, for instance, that biomedicine's inattention to mind-body relations has alienated patients (O'Sullivan, Lipper, and Lerner), while a second set holds that patients consult traditional Chinese medicine due to their "frustration" with biomedicine (Koo and Arain). Dermatologist David Elpern criticizes biomedicine for being obsessed with finding cures for illness at the expense of caring for patients. He argues that patients are attracted to CAM not necessarily because it works but because it addresses their "perceptions of lack of caring evinced by many medical doctors" (1473). Even Tom Delbanco, an outspoken critic of research on CAM, describes biomedicine as a victim of its own success. Ever since the early triumphs of "antibiotic 'miracle drugs' and the polio vaccine" (1560), he maintains, biomedicine has struggled to deliver on its promise of cure, especially for AIDS and cancer. As a result, Delbanco notes, "Public confidence in biomedical science has fallen, and alternative medicine, with its primal message of hope, is currently filling a vacuum" (1560).

Other editorial materials in the *JAMA-Archives* theme issues similarly emphasize that alternative medicine has something to offer patients that

mainstream medicine cannot: individualized attention. This attention becomes an object of praise for many authors in the theme issues, and perhaps
even envy. Although the editorial contributors to the journals are not always
correct in their speculation on why patients seek alternative medicine—
patient dissatisfaction, for example, is not a strong predictor of CAM use (see
Astin)—they nevertheless demonstrate their willingness to think hard about
biomedicine's shortcomings. These contributors recognize, in particular, that
if a patient's well-being is the ultimate outcome measure, then physicians
must consider more than trial data as evidence of an intervention's effect. In
"What Counts as Evidence?" for example, physician Dan Richard recounts
the story of one of his patients who was unmoved by trial evidence that peppermint oil works for headache and could only be persuaded when Richard described his own wife's success with the treatment. In Richard's view,
medical research must ultimately serve practice: "As clinicians, we must ask
ourselves how much evidence is enough to assist patients with their use of
complementary medicines. . . . What about you—does the [randomized controlled trial] evidence convince you to try peppermint oil? Or are you, like my
patient, persuaded more by the testimonial?" (599).

When it comes to actually conducting research on CAM, the *JAMA-
Archives* theme issues tell an altogether different story about evidence. As the
editor of *Archives of Surgery* notes, "in God we trust but everyone else must
have data" (Organ 1153). What counts as "data" in the clinical trial reports and
systematic reviews published in the theme issues is far more restricted than
it is in the editorial materials. While the editorial commentators admit candidly that CAM interventions are popular because they actively attend to
patients' social and psychological needs, those needs are absent in the very
empirical research designed to test the effects of those interventions. The dis-
crepancy between these less and more restrictive perspectives on determining what "works" in CAM returns us to this chapter's central point: although
evidence in medicine is lavishly praised in the abstract, certain kinds of evidence are more praiseworthy in certain contexts than others.

Consider again Taubes's article on hormone-replacement therapy, in
which he indicts all forms of evidence as inherently unreliable but then asserts that the RCT (and only the RCT) can generate the kind of evidence we
can rely on. The slipperiness of data depends partly on context: on their own,
RCTs are rife with problems, but within evidence-based medicine's hierarchies of evidence, they are the best we have got.[6] However, the importance
of the RCT in the production of biomedical evidence is often overestimated,
particularly given that one of evidence-based medicine's founding tenets is
that the highest-level currently *available* evidence is sufficient enough, at that

moment, for a practice to be considered evidence-based—with the proviso, always, that "more evidence is needed."

The problem with RCT-derived evidence on complementary and alternative medicine is that the data are often difficult to interpret and apply in practice. Without an overarching common standard between biomedicine and the CAM interventions under study, triallists must carefully assess the compatibility of their design with both accepted biomedical methodologies and the principles of the intervention under study; when the two do not match up, researchers generally reshape the CAM interventions so that they better fit into a conventional biomedical mold. For example, to meet the biomedical norm of treatment standardization, Shlay et al. invented what they called a "Standardized Acupuncture Regimen" (SAR) to treat HIV-related peripheral neuropathy. This standardized approach meant that all patients from the intervention group received exactly the same acupuncture treatment (needles applied to a fixed set of acupoints) rather than receiving a tailor-made treatment in accordance with the procedures of traditional Chinese medicine (TCM).

Although the SAR was selected by a panel of experienced acupuncturists, the practice as manifest in the study bears little resemblance to its clinical counterpart.[7] During the discourse-based interviews that I conducted for this book, Dr. Yao, the founder and president of a major metropolitan school of TCM, responded to the concept of the SAR with disbelief: "Everybody receives the same point?" He dismissed the form of acupuncture in the study as not even recognizable to him as TCM. The other acupuncturist I interviewed, Dr. Connolly, a Western-born, early-career TCM practitioner specializing in reproductive health, was instead more open, conceptually, to the idea of standardization. He could identify with the quantifying impulse of Western medical culture but likened such an approach in acupuncture to "trying to fit an ocean into a bathtub." (Sounding amused, he said of the SAR, "they think they standardized what I do.")

Not surprisingly, the study's standardized approach is exactly what made this study more credible to the medical researchers I interviewed, Dr. Clarke, then the director of a major hospital-based center for clinical epidemiology and research design, and Dr. Fournier, a junior researcher at the same center. For these researchers, the study's standardized intervention eliminated individual variations in the treatment under study to ensure that each patient received an identical intervention. To approach the study any other way would, to them, compromise its rigor by introducing contaminating variability.

The TCM practitioners I interviewed were also troubled by the Shlay study's methods of blinding, particularly its use of an active placebo control, which placed three needles in locations on the leg that do not correspond to any known acupuncture points. The theory behind the study's active control points was that, because they were not located along any traditional *qi* meridians, the needles should have minimal or no effect and yet maintain participant blinding because needles were visibly inserted into the skin. When I asked Drs. Yao and Connolly about the use of this active control, neither accepted the idea of a placebo effect in traditional Chinese medicine. Both argued that TCM treats a patient's mind and body together as one: if a patient improves, it does not matter in their view whether the treatment's effect was "real" or imaginary.

Yao and Connolly were both willing to go along with the idea of using a placebo control for the sake of our discussion of the Shlay study's methods, but, even still, they worried about the particular methods chosen. Yao was concerned about the use of an active control point, a needle actually inserted into the skin, when, in his view, the triallists could have easily used an inactive control by simply tapping the skin to mimic the sensation of needle insertion. ("That's a mistake," he said. "This is negligent. They didn't think carefully about this.") Connolly was more concerned about the validity of the control points *as* control points, observing that "my intention, as someone treating, matters, so me knowing that I am . . . administering something that isn't going to be effective will affect the treatment." He felt that, without *intention* behind the placebo treatment as an innate healing principle, the procedure would fail to meet the basic requirement of a placebo to be identical in all ways to the study intervention except the active ingredient, in this case, the connection between meridian and needle.[8] Curiously, Connolly's concern stemmed from the fact that the study was not *double-blind*—a concern nested not in the framework of TCM but, instead, in that of evidence-based medicine.

These two examples from the Shlay study, the use of standardization and placebo controls, illustrate how randomized controlled trials in the *JAMA-Archives* theme issues mold CAM practices into a biomedical framework. Both TCM practitioners I interviewed were uncomfortable with the differences between acupuncture as performed in the study and acupuncture as performed in everyday TCM practice, each declaring the trial's results irrelevant to their own care of patients. The medical researchers, by contrast, initially felt that the differences between the intervention in the study and its delivery in TCM practice were insignificant and that the study's methods of standardization and control signaled the researchers' commitment to established scientific procedures. (On further consideration, both researchers changed their minds about the study, as I explain below.)

The other trial I analyze in this chapter, the Cardini and Weixin trial of moxibustion (the burning of herb rolls on acupoints), stands out as an anomaly among the randomized controlled trials in the *JAMA-Archives* CAM-themed issues. While the other RCTs produced mixed but largely negative results, Cardini and Weixin's study showed a strongly positive result of moxibustion's effect on the reversal of breech pregnancies. Its methods and outcomes measures are more consistent with the conventions of biomedical research than the other RCTs in the theme issues: the study intervention was standardized across participants without distorting TCM theory (both TCM practitioners I interviewed agreed that the selected acupoint, BL 67, would singularly be used on all women with breech pregnancies); the placebo arm was genuinely inactive, with placebo-arm participants receiving only routine maternity care, rather than a potentially active control; and outcomes were measured objectively by the research team by determining head position by ultrasound and at birth, whereas most of the other RCTs in the theme issues were assessed by subjective, patient-reported measures such as symptom diaries and pain scores. Despite all of these design features, which struck me as relatively strong, research methodologists Clarke and Fournier both remained skeptical about the study's methods.

Both researchers worried, for example, that some participants might "get more" of the study treatment than others if they have a higher tolerance of burning sensations. They also expressed concern about variability because the treatment was administered at home by nonmedical personnel. Fournier searched even further for possible confounding variables, noting at one point that, "It seems to me, if you can burn stuff on your toes and it makes an influence then a lot of things might be able to influence this breech presentation at this point." Given that Cardini and Weixin do explain in their study that participants were advised to consult the investigators before using "any other interventions or therapies that could contaminate the results of the trial" (1581), Fournier's concern about confounding variables may be more a reflection of his own disposition toward moxibustion than of a flaw in the study's design. Both he and Clarke expressed concern frequently that contamination might have creeped unnoticed into the two acupuncture studies, a worry that I suspect may not have been so pervasive if they were assessing a conventional biomedical study.

Both Clarke and Fournier cited potential variability in application and dosage of moxibustion as a significant flaw in the Cardini and Weixin trial, while they commended the use of standardization and placebo controls in the Shlay study. In each case, these expert readers isolated individual elements of an idealized RCT model and measured the acupuncture trials against them. However, as Clarke and Fournier later reflected further on the validity and applicability of the studies' findings, both reevaluated their own initial responses to the studies' design. For example, although Clarke had earlier praised standardization as one of the Shlay study's "very positive features," when he realized that the standardized acupuncture regimen did not reflect or apply to actual TCM practice, he determined that standardization was ultimately not essential to the quality of the design. He offered this comparison:

> If you were giving a psychotherapy intervention, let's say, there'd be some sort of flexibility in terms of the approach you would take. There'd be some individualization of that treatment, I can understand this. But if you believe that these [energy] pathways are real and the people are trained to identify those pathways, it shouldn't [pose a problem], I guess. I'd turn the comment around and say, "Well you should design a randomized trial where you do a personalized intervention versus sham and then see what happens."

In suggesting that an individualized treatment would not alone compromise the integrity of a trial—particularly since, as he notes, individualization is also routine in some biomedical trials—Clarke has shifted his criteria here for what counts as an appropriate methodology. At first, standardization served as a firm benchmark for determining the quality of the Shlay study but, as the study's larger context and implications became clearer to him, it became less important.

This example shows that, in biomedical boundary work, standards that are held up as benchmarks of accepted methodologies, such as randomization and placebo controls, are often more flexible than they initially seem. Although standardization is certainly conventional in biomedicine, it is by no means essential to trial design—nursing and psychotherapy trials, for example, frequently feature individualized interventions without compromising the quality of their evidence. The Shlay study's adoption of a standardized regimen despite that regimen's irrelevance to practice (1594) therefore signals that something larger than concern for methodological integrity may be at work in the study's design. Examining how researchers such as Shlay et al. and Cardini and Weixin design their studies of interventions that do not fit easily into the RCT framework betrays the researchers' awareness of the need to fit their study within the expected norms of biomedical research. However, their efforts to meet particular standards of evidence also reveal the potential for method to serve argumentative ends in biomedical boundary work because, as I show next, the randomized controlled trial is an idealized model that, even in mainstream medicine, frequently falls short of its reputation as the "gold standard."

Idealizing Research: The Genre of the
Randomized Controlled Trial Report

In biomedical boundary work, genres of professional publication help to determine the limits of what counts as evidence for a given health practice and what does not. The genre of the randomized controlled trial report, in particular, is a key constituent of the method topos in debates about complementary and alternative medicine. All of the RCT reports in the *JAMA-Archives* theme issues follow the IMRaD structure (introduction, methods, results, and discussion) recommended by the International Committee of Medical Journal Editors in the uniform requirements for manuscripts submitted to biomedical journals. Modeled on the genre of the experimental article borrowed from the sciences, this format serves specific and recurrent rhetorical purposes because it does not just sort information into clearly defined categories—more importantly, the RCT report transforms the knowledge it produces and the communities that use it. As a genre, the RCT report enforces biomedical boundaries because it embodies an idealized model of research that seems, from the start, to set up the testing of CAM for failure.

The authors of both acupuncture trials at the center of this chapter appear strategically to employ the genre of the RCT report to enhance their ethos as scientists in the face of their work on subjects not fully compatible with a biomedical purview. In the Shlay study, for instance, the article's arrangement in the IMRaD structure helps to downplay the strangeness of traditional Chinese medical theory within biomedicine as well as the study's incompatibility with that theory. When the authors first mention their standardized approach in their introduction, the procedure is simply asserted, without contextualization, and is easy to miss:

> To evaluate the effect of both a nonstandard and standard medical therapy for peripheral neuropathy, we performed a multicenter, modified double-blind, randomized, placebo-controlled study of the separate and combined efficacy of a standardized acupuncture regimen (SAR) and amitriptyline for the relief of pain caused by HIV-related peripheral neuropathy. (1590)

None of the expert readers I interviewed—TCM practitioners Yao and Connolly, researchers Clarke and Fournier, and Dr. McDonald, a midcareer family physician specializing in obstetrical care—even registered this first occurrence of the SAR as a textual entity. Each participant asked what a "SAR" was when the term came up again later in the article. Shlay et al.'s article does not explain until the final discussion section why the intervention was standardized or that standardization is incompatible with TCM practice, even though all five expert readers felt that this background information was pertinent to their assessment of the study's methods and results.

Given that introductions and discussions are the sections of experimental articles that scientists are the least likely to read (Berkenkotter and Huckin), the fact that Shlay et al. only contextualize or explain the SAR within these peripheral discursive spaces, leaving the term otherwise unexplained, minimizes their study's association with traditional Chinese medicine as an independent professional and philosophical practice. In the methods and results sections, the authors abstract needling out of traditional Chinese medicine and present it à la carte as "SAR," without any guiding theory or context. McDonald, the physician-clinician I interviewed, was surprised to learn at the end of the article, in the discussion section, that the study intervention varied so markedly from TCM practice: "That's helpful, because I wouldn't have inferred that."

Within the framework of Ellen Prince's linguistic-pragmatic taxonomy of assumed familiarity, the SAR's initial appearance following an indefinite article—"*a* standardized acupuncture regimen (SAR)"—introduces the SAR as a "brand new" textual entity (235), something presumed not to be familiar within a particular discourse community. In this case, the SAR is framed as outside the medical community's shared store of knowledge. (Amitriptyline, by contrast, is a named entity introduced with a definite expression, assumed to be familiar to medical readers.) The next time the SAR is mentioned, in the methods section, the authors explain only how they selected the acupoints, and not that the selected approach varies from typical acupuncture practice. All subsequent references simply invoke the SAR as an already familiar concept, so that readers must search back in the text to find the original reference in the introduction to discern its meaning. Given how little time medical personnel have available to keep up with the clinical trial literature generally (Grimes and Schulz; Sackett et al.), it seems unlikely that any but the most interested readers would go searching back in the text to find the initial definition of the SAR. I suspect that such readers would, instead, do as Clarke, Fournier, and McDonald did, and simply take the SAR as an uncontroversial given.[9]

When Shlay et al. do discuss the SAR at the article's end, they explain its divergence from practice matter-of-factly: "The SAR chosen for this study differs from the practice of most acupuncturists, who treat patients with individualized regimens" (1594). In this statement, the authors' reference to "the SAR chosen" is what Prince calls a "containing inferrable" (236), a textual entity whose meaning is inferrable from the statement itself. A reader asking, of this statement, "Which SAR are the authors referring to?" could answer, "Oh, the one chosen in the study." Although this statement—"the SAR chosen"—is circular in its reference, in that it provides within itself the resources for its own interpretation, this construction also implies that SARs are generally an established category. Phrased this way, it sounds almost as though Shlay et al. are explaining why they chose *this* SAR over another one.

The placement of explanatory information about the SAR within peripheral sections of the IMRaD structure therefore helps to emphasize the Shlay study's alignment with biomedical conventions by distancing it from acupuncture theory and practice. The authors situate their study more squarely in the bounds of biomedicine by explaining in the discussion that, in selecting their standardized study intervention, they prioritized blinding, replication, and generalizability of results over fidelity to the principles of acupuncture as it is performed in TCM practice. Further, by emphasizing the study's alignment with biomedical principles, the article deflects attention from its inability to argue from the topos of external consistency (Prelli), a characteristic rhetorical strategy in scientific articles that allows scientific authors to demonstrate the consistency of their current claims with the established, common store of knowledge of their field. Shlay et al. are unable to make such claims because their standardized intervention is not consistent with acupuncture as it is performed in practice.

Although acupuncture theory would not be considered part of the store of shared knowledge in science, the fact that the study's SAR was not consistent even with the traditional Chinese medical community's own agreed-upon rules of practice was not lost on my researcher-readers Clarke and Fournier, perhaps because it violated a more expansive principle of consistency, in their view. Fournier, for example, noted that although Shlay et al. were seeking reproducible results by choosing a standardized intervention, "we always want to do things that reflect practice, right? So the fact that this doesn't reflect practice . . . [means] this is of very little relevance, the results." Even still, although both researchers ultimately questioned the strength and significance of the evidence produced by the Shlay study, we should not lose sight of the fact that each was initially impressed by the study's design and only came to view it differently after extended discussion of specific passages within the article. More casual readers of these articles—time-strapped researchers and clinicians— may not move far beyond these readers' initial impressions, which were shaped by the genre of the RCT report itself. In the *JAMA-Archives* theme issues, the genre of the RCT report enhances the studies' legitimacy within biomedicine because the conventions of that genre align studies of complementary and alternative medicine with biomedical ways of thinking and acting.

We know from genre theory, particularly from Carolyn Miller's seminal formulation of genres as "typified rhetorical actions based in recurrent situations" ("Genre" 159), that genres accomplish important rhetorical work: genres shape the production of discourses and condition their reception; genres are instrumental in processes of identification, notably in academic and professional settings where writers must demonstrate their mastery of their field's genres to assert their community membership and establish themselves as authorities; and genres perform important epistemic functions, both in the discourses they enact and among the discourse communities that use them. Berkenkotter and Huckin note that "Genres are intimately linked to a discipline's methodology, and they package information in ways that conform to a discipline's norms, values, and ideology" (1)—genres are, in short, "the intellectual scaffolds on which community-based knowledge is constructed" (24).

Genres can be difficult to isolate and describe, however, because, as Anthony Paré explains, "The automatic, ritual unfolding of genres makes them appear normal, even inevitable; they are simply the way things are done" (59). This sense of generic "inevitability" lends itself to a sort of generic *invisibility*, particularly in science, a world shaped by genres meant to disappear. Scientific articles, for example, seem to leave readers with only objective facts. But, despite their seeming objectivity, genres embody unconscious, tacit social actions, and so are inherently ideological. In science, that ideology inheres in its institutionalized genres—grant proposals, lab reports, conference papers, experimental articles, and so on.

In medicine, the RCT report, modeled on the genre of the experimental article in science, is one of its central intellectual scaffolds, the structure through which medicine's most valued forms of evidence are produced. But the application of the genre of the experimental article to medicine is uneasy. As much as the RCT report seems to affirm biomedicine's standing as a scientific enterprise, historian of science Theodore Porter explains that the "relative rigidity" of the rules about conducting and publishing experiments and their results (i.e., the IMRaD model) instead "ought to be understood in part as a way of generating a shared discourse, of unifying a weak research community" (228). For Porter, weak communities are simply those, such as medicine and psychology, that rely on science but are not themselves singularly scientific: "Scientific knowledge is most likely to display conspicuously the trappings of science in fields with insecure borders, communities with persistent boundary problems. . . . Some of the most distinctive and typical features of scientific discourse reflect this weakness of community" (230).

Following on Porter's argument, the adoption of the IMRaD model in medicine could be seen as a persuasive move on the community level, where the users of the genre actively (though not necessarily consciously) foster identification between their methods and the valorized methods of science in order to secure their community's boundaries and their position within them. This anxiety is particularly intense in the discourse of evidence-based medicine, which frequently frames the need for greater production and consumption of evidence not as a matter of medicine becoming more scientific but of catching up with the *other* disciplines of science. Note, for example, the tenor of physician-researcher R. M. Califf's admonishment in the *Journal of Internal Medicine* in 2003: "The failure of the medical professions to develop and implement data standards has left medicine far behind most other major enterprises" (427).

Other fields of study have also capitalized on the mobilizing force of the scientific article, particularly the social sciences. More than half a century ago, rhetoric scholar Richard Weaver observed that the methods of science had been so successful at formulating knowledge claims that researchers in other disciplines, such as sociology, began to apply the generic features of scientific articles to their own disciplines. In adopting these features, Weaver explained, researchers "were not trying to state the nature of their subject; they were trying to get a value imputed to it" (143). The value associated with scientific genres can be understood as a form of linguistic capital, in Pierre Bourdieu's terms, because the discourses of science have come to be "worth" more in research culture than other discourses. In this view, disciplines that sit on the edges of science, or beyond them, may import scientific genres into their own forms of communication as a means of fostering identification with science and its attendant linguistic capital. This "borrowing" of scientific genres is part of the communally instantiated action of genre within research culture.[10]

The notion of genre-borrowing is salient to the acupuncture trials I examine in this chapter. Although the Shlay et al. and Cardini and Weixin articles are ostensibly in the biomedical mainstream, authored by established biomedical researchers and published under the imprimatur of the American Medical Association, they can also usefully be thought of as borrowed genres: they apply the habits of mind and modes of communication of one field (medicine) to another disparate, possibly incommensurate field (acupuncture). In the genre of the RCT report, then, the terministic screen of experimental science "directs the attention" (Burke, *Language* 45) of researchers toward observations about acupuncture that fit that experimental terminology and away from others that do not. For example, in the Shlay study, the IMRaD format directs attention away from the more idiosyncratic elements of acupuncture in TCM because there appears to be no room in that genre for concepts such as *qi* or *meridians*, for individualized therapies, or, indeed, for nonstandardized approaches to health, generally.[11]

Perhaps not surprisingly, then, both the Cardini and Weixin and the Shlay articles exhibit a kind of hyperperformance of the experimental genre as they "display conspicuously the trappings of science" (T. Porter). Most strikingly, both articles assume an exaggerated empiricity, an overdescription of salient trial features that increase the studies' association with scientific methods. This overdescription struck my expert readers as a little suspect. Physician-clinician McDonald, for example, was mystified by Cardini and Weixin's instructions to the study's participants regarding how to sense, at home, whether reversal of the fetus' breech position had occurred. She spent nearly five minutes of the interview working through this one description of what patients should watch for: "decreased pressure in the epigastrium or hypochondrium, increased pressure in the hypogastrium, pollakiuria, [or] a 'different feeling' in the abdomen" (1581). Mapping on her own body where these different sensations would be felt, McDonald struggled to understand them:

> I just read that and I thought, "Okay that's the same area, I don't know why they are saying it twice" and then "increased pressure in the hypogastrium"— honestly, I had a hard time literally trying to imagine what they meant by that and I thought "uh?" 'Cause as far as I can tell on my own body, your epigastrium, right up here by your tummy, so "decrease pressure there," okay, but then they're saying, well, on the other hand, you might have more pressure like, seriously, two inches below it and I thought, "Okay?" I didn't know what they meant by that.

McDonald noted that since even she, as a physician, had a hard time distinguishing between the different sensations described, she did not feel that such a minutely detailed description of symptoms would be a useful "clinical clue to women to . . . keep an eye out for."

McDonald also found the description of trial features and effects in Cardini and Weixin's study to be unusually technical in its description. For example, she was unfamiliar with terms such as "pollakiuria," in the passage above, and others elsewhere, such as "gestosis," each of which refers to common clinical presentations—in this case, excessive urination and preeclampsia. Given that McDonald encounters both conditions regularly in her practice and yet was unfamiliar with either of these terms, Cardini and Weixin's use of these specialized terms to describe ordinary bodily states suggested to her that the authors were trying to strengthen their article's ties to the scientific community. She responded similarly to the study's outcomes measures, which included not only cephalic (head-first) presentation at 35 weeks' gestation and at birth but also fetal motor activity, adverse events, cephalic versions, caesarean sections, spontaneous and induced deliveries, and Apgar scores. Considering that the study examined interventions for reversal of breech presentation, Mc-Donald felt that the authors' inclusion of outcomes beyond head-first delivery "seemed, if anything, overly comprehensive," as if the authors were "trying to make [their article] sound more slick" by overdescribing simple concepts in complex scientific terms.

This sense of overdescription runs through both articles, but I would argue that it is a *strategic* overdescription, aimed at persuasion. In the Shlay study, for example, the explicitly detailed description of the needle insertion protocol is most revealing in what it does not say:

> For the SAR and control points, acupuncture needles were inserted to a specified depth. Each location was manipulated both superiorly and inferiorly. Then the needles were reinserted into the specified point. After 10 to 15 minutes, the needles were remanipulated and replaced into the original location for another 5 to 10 minutes. The depth of insertion was between 1.28 to 2.54 cm (0.5 to 1.0 in) for spleen point 9, 2.54 to 3.81 cm (1.0 to 1.5 in) for spleen point 7, and 1.5 to 3.05 cm (0.6 to 1.2 in) for spleen point 6. For the control points, insertion was less than 1.28 cm (0.5 in). (1591)

The traditional Chinese medicine practitioners I interviewed struggled to understand the manipulation technique described in this passage. "I don't understand this little portion," Connolly said. "I really read it, like, four times to get it and I can't." Yao reread the description aloud to himself several times while manipulating imaginary acupuncture needles in the air in front of him. Both practitioners wondered: Why would the needles need to be reinserted? Why would they be removed at all? What is superior manipulation? How were the depths determined?

Although Shlay et al. describe the needle manipulation protocol in painstaking detail—in so much detail that my study acupuncturists could not even keep track of its specificity—there is no description, in this passage or elsewhere, about *why* the needles need to manipulated. The meridian theory of acupuncture to enable the flow of *qi* is conspicuously absent in the Shlay study. The authors gesture toward an underlying mechanism in the discussion, but their explanation is strictly biochemical: "mechanisms such as the release of endogenous opioids or activation of other brain and spinal cord pathways that reduce pain" (1594). The absence in the methods section of any underlying theory regarding the intervention's mechanism of action makes the authors' careful description of the needle manipulation protocol seem strangely undermotivated. Indeed, both Fournier, the medical researcher, and McDonald, the physician-clinician, seemed bemused by the level of detail given, a bemusement that appeared to stem from the article's lack of reasoning behind the complicated needle routine.

In considering the rhetorical dimensions of biomedical boundary work, the key question in this example is: Why do the authors describe the needle manipulation protocol so carefully but not give any explanation regarding why the procedure was performed that way? Rhetorically, one answer is that this description-without-explanation downplays the study's association with traditional Chinese medicine as an independent professional and philosophical practice. And yet this description seems also to serve another purpose, one that addresses the premium placed in biomedicine on *method*—the means to knowledge, as Kaptchuk notes ("Powerful"), rather than knowledge itself. Method is one of the primary ways that scientists identify themselves as members of their intellectual and professional communities and persuade readers to take their results seriously. In boundary disputes, method can be invoked rhetorically to position a given health practice within or beyond the borders of science.

Method as a Boundary Argument

In biomedical research on complementary and alternative medicine, emphasizing a study's adherence to scientific methods helps to align trials of boundary-crossing health practices with biomedicine's community-defined norms, values, and procedures. From this perspective, it makes sense that Shlay et al. frame their methods in a scientific lexicon to the point of overdescription, describing needle depths to one-hundredths of a millimeter, and yet avoid altogether the concept of *qi* as a mechanism of action in the intervention. Any discussion of a "life force" that moves along traditional Chinese meridians would undermine the authors' credibility as scientists, since neither *qi* nor meridians have ever been scientifically demonstrated to exist. Without that credibility, their study could not be validated as a legitimate contribution to the biomedical community's store of knowledge.

The problem with such emphasis on method in biomedical research on CAM is that the chances of an intervention such as acupuncture meeting the methodological standards enacted by the IMRaD format *while* remaining consonant with the core tenets of its own philosophical system, traditional Chinese medicine, *and* demonstrating a measurable effect are poor indeed. And yet, importantly, the genre of the clinical trial report idealizes standards of evidence that even biomedical studies frequently fail to meet. Given this context, I argue in this section that, in debates about CAM, we can read demands that CAM meet the same (or even stricter) standards of evidence as indicative of higher-order concerns in the medical profession about its own methods of study and practice.

Linguist and genre scholar John Swales observes that "the fact that the purposes of some genres may be hard to get at is itself of considerable heuristic value" (46). This is where the real ideological work of genres comes into play, particularly in science and medicine, where genres seem only to serve the purpose of providing information. The IMRaD structure, for instance, appears to facilitate the objective reporting of the events and implications of a given research project, wherein authors "writing up" their results "seem only to be contributing a filler for a defined slot" (Bazerman, *Shaping Written Knowledge* 28).[12] However, despite its apparent neutrality, the IMRaD structure itself explicitly embodies certain systemic values about scientific knowledge that are central to science's position of privilege in Western culture.

Central to this embodied value system is the idealized model of research that emerges through it: real-life science evolves more organically, more accidentally, than the IMRaD model would suggest. Experimental reports, unlike their correspondent laboratory and clinical notes, adopt a more solution-oriented stance and divide the various, overlapping elements of research practice into finite sections. The notes are not just "written up"—they are reordered, and their levels and kinds of claims are altered, their emphases shifted, and their vocabularies adapted to meet specific goals, which often vary markedly from the initial goals of the project (Swales 117–27). This was the warrant for Nobel Prize-winning medical researcher Peter Medawar's claim in 1964 that the genre of the scientific paper is "fraudulent," because it "misrepresents" scientific processes.

Methods sections of experimental articles in science and medicine exist ostensibly for the sake of replication, to enable other researchers to repeat a study's methods to confirm or discount its findings. Shlay et al., for instance, explicitly cite replication as one of main motives behind their standardized regimen. In actual research practice, however, methods sections are often poorly suited to duplication because they are so "elliptical" in their phrasing that their procedures are not explicit enough for other researchers to follow (Swales 169). Furthermore, there is little incentive within science to replicate studies, since the rewards of science go to innovation, to studies that break new ground rather than simply reinvestigate familiar terrain (Collins; Gilbert and Mulkay). When scientists do wish to replicate a study, they generally reframe their replication so that it constitutes something new, rather than "mere" replication (Gilbert and Mulkay). Given their abstractness, therefore, methods sections in experimental articles seem primarily to serve persuasive ends, to shore up a study's scientific authority. They do so, I argue, by working as arguments from both *prolepsis*—anticipating and heading off objections by indicating the appropriateness of the study's methodology—and *ethos*— enhancing the researcher's character *qua* researcher. Accordingly, I argue, the emphasis on methodology in experimental articles is significant less because it makes research replicable than simply because it makes research recognizable as scientific.[13]

The genre of the RCT report fixes an ideal of research that most CAM practices cannot meet, particularly not in an evidence-based model. In evidence-based medicine, data derived from randomized controlled trials and from meta-analysis of multiple trials comprise the gold standard, while data produced by methods lower on the evidence hierarchy, such as unblinded studies or case reports, fail to achieve that standard. Given the methodological problems associated with testing practices such as acupuncture in randomized controlled trials, the consequent shortage of evidence of their efficacy is often taken as "evidence of the lack of an effect" (Stener-Victorin et al. 1942). The dismissal of CAM on such grounds, in which commentators invoke stricter or looser interpretations of what constitutes a valid methodology or valid evidence depending on their own political and ideological orientation, shares some parallels with arguments in areas of what Ceccarelli calls "manufactured controversy" in science, such as climate change, intelligent design, and Big Tobacco (Ceccarelli, "Manufactured"; Michaels; Oreskes and Conway).

Contributors to the *JAMA-Archives* theme issues on CAM are able to invoke varying standards of evidence production to limit or expand biomedicine's scope and the place of complementary and alternative medicine within it. For example, in the *JAMA* theme issue, Tom Delbanco views CAM as an imminent threat to the medical profession; he also demands much higher standards of evidence production than did Clarke, one of the medical researchers that I interviewed, who was unconcerned about the prospect of CAM encroaching on biomedicine. Whereas Delbanco dismisses CAM research because of difficulties of controlling for CAM's interactive and placebo effects, Clarke accepted the idiosyncrasies of such research. Remaining alert to matters of scientific protocol, Clarke was willing, for example, to consider the similar design problems that some biomedical studies face, such as those on psychotherapeutic interventions, which I discussed earlier in this chapter.

If we situate the debate about CAM occurring in the *JAMA-Archives* theme issues within the larger context of evidence-based medicine, we can more carefully highlight the role of method in boundary-negotiating arguments. Although the literature on evidence-based medicine has valorized the randomized controlled trial, it has, at the same time, fostered a thriving culture of critique of both EBM's methods and its ideology. These critiques helpfully illuminate the RCT's uneven ability to demonstrate the safety and efficacy of health interventions, as well as illuminate the RCT's own "self-authenticating logic."[14] For example, sociologist Catherine Will has examined "the ways in which modifications of the 'pure' world of the experiment may also be seen as strengthening the evidence it is intended to produce" (85). Referring to this strengthening process as the "alchemy" of the clinical trial, she notes that the various contingencies of research—the many different sorts of people, technologies, institutions, funding bodies, and more involved in a particular project—are transformed, in part through "the ritual invocation of random-ization and control," into objective, hard facts about the world (97).

Clinical trial evidence is reified through this process of transformation, where it is framed no longer as an *ideal* of research but as a necessary and always attainable framework for producing valid knowledge about human health. The editors of the *JAMA-Archives* theme issues, Fontanarosa and Lund-berg, accordingly set the bar of evidence production high when they describe what they believe to be the theme issues' primary outcome:

> these investigat[ions] demonstrate that alternative medicine therapies and in-terventions can and should be evaluated using explicit, focused research ques-tions along with established and accepted rigorous research methods (e.g., appropriate controls, effective blinding procedures, adequate power, state-of-the-art techniques for systematic reviews); incorporating measurable, objec-tively assessed end points (e.g., blinded assessment); and reporting meaningful patient-centered outcomes. ("Alternative Medicine" 1619)

Fontanarosa and Lundberg seem unaware of the deep ironies of their claims. Most immediately, the methods of (at least) the studies examined in this chapter fail to meet the standards that the editors claim for the theme issues as a whole. For example, both of the research methodologists I interviewed, Fournier and Clarke, cited serious problems with the studies' ethics, random-ization, standardization, blinding, statistical power, and outcomes assessment. Each researcher expressed surprise that the two studies were published in *JAMA* at all, given these problems. When I informed them at the end of their interviews that the articles were part of a theme issue on CAM, both research-ers surmised that the articles were likely published only because, in their view, theme issues have lower standards for acceptance than regular journal issues.

The second and bigger irony of Fontanarosa and Lundberg's characteriza-tion of the clinical trials within theme issue is that, despite their proleptic in-sistence that the CAM trials were evaluated according to the same standards as biomedical trials, biomedicine itself routinely fails those standards. In an early critique of evidence-based medicine from 1997, for example, Yale medical researchers Feinstein and Horwitz argued that less than half of the studies analyzed in a review of methodological quality had met basic scientific standards (533). Similarly, other critics have isolated blinding (e.g., Fergusson et al.), randomization (Chalmers), assessment scales (Jüni et al.), and placebo controls (Lakoff) as key areas of weakness in biomedical research. More recently, in 2015, Ben Goldacre and Carl Heneghan published in the *British Medical Journal* a blistering critique of the current state of biomedical evidence, which they argue is marred by weak outcomes measures, publication bias, industry sponsorship (which overwhelming produces the results desired by study sponsors), and more. (See also Angell, who argues that nearly every aspect of biomedical research is suspect, particularly in pharmaceutical trials.)

Critiques of evidence-based medicine are useful to the study of boundary work in biomedical research on CAM because they point to a deeply penetrating instability in the evidence base. This instability can largely be traced back to the clinical trial report as one of EBM's organizing genres. In a 2004 critique of evidence-based medicine, for example, physician Abd Hamid Mat Sain dismissed EBM's reliance on the RCT as "the panaceal standard bearer of evidence." Several years prior, in 2001, Ted Kaptchuk similarly wondered aloud if the RCT really is the gold standard, or if it is, instead, a "golden calf" ("Double-Blind"). Even psychiatrist Simon Wessely, who passionately defends the RCT in mental health trials, avers that it "is not the pot of gold at the end of the evidence-based rainbow" (116).

In Fontanarosa and Lundberg's opening statement in their *JAMA* editorial, which I quoted at the beginning of chapter 1, the editors invoke a binary between "proven" and "unproven" medicine: proven medicine, they say, is evidence-based, while unproven medicine lacks evidence. In this configuration, biomedicine falls under the first category, while interventions such as acupuncture fall under the second, although ostensibly with the potential to move into the first category after adequate testing. While this proven-unproven binary holds an intuitive logic, it works less as a legitimate claim about the conditions of knowledge-making in medicine than as a straw man argument when we consider that the majority of biomedical treatments have also not been proven according to these same criteria (Borgerson).

Given that biomedical studies so regularly do not achieve the same standards to which CAM studies are held, we might instead usefully think of Fontanarosa and Lundberg's distinction between proven and unproven therapies as a reflection of the *symbolic* value that the randomized controlled trial holds in medicine, as representative of the aims and ideals of research rather than as a true characterization of research culture as it actually exists. This is how the rhetorical study of research on complementary and alternative medicine can illuminate biomedicine itself, by opening up its evidentiary methods to scrutiny through a kind of Brechtian alienation—that is, by making them "strange."

It is not just the randomized controlled trial's claims to rigor that are problematic, however: its relevance, too, is often hard to demonstrate. For example, Fontanarosa and Lundberg assume that adequate testing will ensure the safety and efficacy of any medical treatment applied in practice, alternative or otherwise, but that assumption is also faulty. We know that there is a poor association between the evidence base and clinical behavior (Denis et al.; Dopson et al.; Grimes and Schulz; Will). Some researchers characterize that weak association as an "implementation gap," where practitioners simply lag behind their research counterparts (see Will), while others see it as the product of a more fundamental mismatch between the theory and practice of medicine (Feinstein and Horwitz).

Part of the disconnection between research and practice certainly has to do with practitioners' ability to keep up with the literature. Sackett et al. report, for example, that doctors have less than an hour per week available to literature review (McDonald reported having less than an hour per *month*), while Grimes and Schulz indicate that many doctors even "feel unqualified" to read the literature "critically" (57). Additionally, the assumption that research findings would so directly translate into practice naively underestimates the complex negotiations that clinicians must undertake among competing bodies of data (RCT reports and systematic reviews, experience, professional habits and competition, commercial interests, clinical practice guidelines, insurance schemes, patient preferences . . .).

An even greater problem with the usefulness of clinical trial results is that, to meet the required standards of internal consistency, trials must sacrifice their external consistency—philosopher of science Nancy Cartwright calls this the problem of "front-end rigour vs. back-end rigour" (19). Cartwright's reasoning is worth quoting in full:

> An argument that certain procedures achieve a given result much of the time may not be a good argument that they do so on any one occasion. External validity for RCTs is hard to justify. Other methods, less rigorous at the front end, on internal validity, can have far better warrant at the back end, on external validity. We must be careful about the trade-offs. There is no a priori reason to

favour a method that is rigorous part of the way and very iffy thereafter over one that reverses the order or one that is less rigorous but fairly well reasoned throughout. (19)

The focus on internal consistency limits the clinical relevance of many studies because the selection criteria are so restricted and the trial populations so homogeneous that the results are difficult to extrapolate to general populations. Health services researcher Nick Black, for instance, found that one trial of coronary bypass had such rigid inclusion criteria that 96 percent of those currently receiving the intervention would not have qualified in the original trials (Bensing 19). So, ultimately, what we know from clinical trial data about a given health intervention is limited to its effects on a small, unnaturally uniform subset of its potential patient population. If we reframe this issue in rhetorical terms, conventional arguments in scientific and medical research that draw on the topos of external consistency may, in some cases, be little more than exercises in argumentation.

Much of the art of medical research lies in striking an appropriate balance between front-end rigor and back-end rigor for a specific research question, to make the results as accurate as possible (i.e., internally valid) but also as useful as possible (i.e., externally valid). Because a study's validity depends on factors such as whether internal or external consistency are prioritized, what it means to call a given health intervention "effective" is largely a product of rhetorical negotiation, particularly when medicine's boundaries are up for negotiation. I turn to this final point next.

Efficacy as a Boundary Object

Efficacy, and its sister term, *safety*, are cited, mantra-like, throughout the medical literature as the chief focus of research—we want to know which health behaviors and interventions are going to help us and not hurt us. (Cost-effectiveness is a third, but later, concern.[15]) In evidence-based medicine, clear determinations of safety and efficacy are assumed to be the natural and necessary outcomes of research, as Sackett et al. claim: "External clinical evidence both invalidates previously accepted diagnostic tests and treatments and replaces them with new ones that are *more powerful, more accurate, more efficacious*, and *safer*" (72; emphasis added).

These two terms, safety and efficacy, are the primary touchstones for determining the legitimacy of health interventions, particularly regarding complementary and alternative medicine, because they provide the terms of the debate and they condition its outcome. Note, for example, the assertion of the *JAMA-Archives* theme issue editors that "There is no alternative medicine," only proven and unproven medicine. They conclude that "as believers in science and evidence, we must focus on fundamental issues [such as] the need for convincing data on safety and therapeutic efficacy" (Fontanarosa and Lundberg, "Alternative Medicine" 1618). The implication in their claim, as I have suggested in previous chapters, is that if a CAM practice is proven safe and effective, it will be integrated seamlessly into biomedical practice. This reasoning sounds simple enough, but it just is not the case, in part because the determination of whether or not an intervention "works"—its efficacy— is more elastic, more idiosyncratic, than the discourse of evidence-based medicine would suggest. Efficacy is a concept that can be manipulated to make an intervention appear to work, or not.

In this final section, I show how, in biomedical debates about CAM, researchers employ a variable principle of efficacy to reconcile their own disciplinary allegiances with both accepted scientific methodologies and the practices under study. I maintain that, in arguments from the topos of method, the notion of efficacy functions as a rhetorically mobile boundary object that both enables research across disparate fields and can be used strategically, even if unconsciously, to advance certain persuasive ends. This claim shifts into a rhetorical framework Susan Leigh Star and James Griesemer's well-known definition of a boundary object as "an analytic concept of those scientific objects which both inhabit several intersecting social worlds . . . *and* satisfy the informational requirements of each of them" (393; original emphasis). In debates about biomedical boundaries, the notion of efficacy, as a boundary object, holds a persuasive potential that merits further investigation.

In developing their concept of the boundary object, Star and Griesemer examined how, in the development of the multidisciplinary Berkeley Museum of Vertebrate Zoology, divergent groups of actors, both professional and amateur, scientific and administrative, were able to sufficiently reconcile their various and often conflicting perspectives to enable cooperation. Star and Griesemer attributed this ability to the stakeholders' exchange of numerous classes of boundary objects, such as record-keeping practices and standardized artifact indexing, that served different ideological and practical purposes for each category of actors but permitted functional cooperation across them. For Star and Griesemer, the common structure of such objects is sufficiently accessible within "more than one world to make them recognizable, a means of translation. . . . across intersecting social worlds" (393).

Numerous scholars have since taken up the boundary object concept and reframed it: for Joan Fujimura, it becomes part of the "standardized package," an idea that both facilitates work across collectives (which she says boundary objects are good at) and stabilizes facts (which she says they are not good at); whereas for Greg Wilson and Carl Herndl, the boundary object becomes a "rhetorical exigence" that leads to the integration, rather than the demarcation, of social-professional boundaries. The multidisciplinary situations that both Fujimura and Wilson and Herndl describe depend on the actors' sincere interest in collaboration and a sense of mutual respect, even for members of groups historically ranked lower than the others.

For CAM research, the principle of efficacy unites the researchers and enables their work, but the situation itself is not always marked by a sense of equality. Even for those biomedical researchers that work earnestly with CAM practitioners, their relative hierarchies remain always on the horizon and the principle of efficacy they invoke at a particular moment can either unite or divide those involved, depending on the researchers' orientation. For example, for a given trial outcome, an acupuncturist might see the successful demonstration of a clinical effect while a biomedical researcher might instead see nothing but a placebo effect. In weighing the evidence, the biomedical perspective will likely tip the scale in the determining whether or not a given health intervention is effective.

As keywords, *safety* and *efficacy* are flexible enough in medical discourse that they can function as gatekeepers: if an intervention meets one implied standard of efficacy, for example, skeptics can (and often do) invoke a more rigorous, and more exclusive, meaning. This is similar to consensus-denial in arguments about climate change, intelligent design, and Big Tobacco, and to data-engineering in pharmaceutical research, where clinical trial reports can be manipulated to amplify certain of a drug's effects and to downplay others. Within debates about CAM, these terms, "safety" and "efficacy," therefore function as god-terms, in Kenneth Burke's formulation: powerful, indeterminate terms that "[sum] up a manifold of particulars under a single head" (*Religion* 2). (*Freedom* and *love* are quintessential god-terms.) As summary terms, "safety" and "efficacy" carry within them various, and even conflicting, interpretations; they contain, Burke would say, the resources of ambiguity (*Grammar* xix), the fertile ground for persuasion. In biomedicine, the notion of efficacy is ambiguous enough that the question of whether a CAM practice "works" depends very much on whom you ask, what their criteria are, and what the consequences are of their answering.

Within the *JAMA-Archives* theme issues, even those authors who are friendly to the idea of biomedical research on CAM argue that studies of CAM ought to be held to the highest possible standards of evidence within biomedicine. For some of these authors, invoking such high standards is strategic, a means of gaining acceptance for research on interventions that fall beyond biomedicine's boundaries. For example, Margolin, Avants, and Kleber assert in their *JAMA* editorial on problems of research design in CAM studies that "The validity and credibility of alternative medicine investigations will be enhanced by using research designs that embody the highest standards for demonstration of efficacy" (1627). They argue that the only way to quell the "controversy" in medicine surrounding CAM and to counter the "outright skepticism" about individual CAM practices is to employ research designs that are essentially airtight (1626–27). In their view, researchers who wish to produce credible research on CAM must, for example, adopt adequate controls and objective outcomes measures and reduce possible expectation, or placebo, effects.

In considering the notion of evidence as a boundary object with rhetorical mobility, still more significant are arguments that draw subtler links between research design and quality of evidence, such as distinctions between trials of efficacy and of effectiveness. To an outsider, these forms of randomized controlled trial may be indistinguishable. However, the difference is crucial in evidence-based medicine, where "current best evidence" has come to mean, almost exclusively, evidence obtained through efficacy studies. These studies feature rigid inclusion criteria, homogeneous participant populations, and, ideally, unambiguous endpoints to minimize statistical "noise." Efficacy studies consequently have high internal validity but possibly limited applicability to real-life populations. (In Cartwright's terminology, they have high front-end rigor but low back-end rigor.) In contrast, effectiveness studies are large, community-based studies of more heterogeneous groups, which trade methodological fastidiousness for applicability in what health care management researcher Steve Maguire calls the "real-world messiness" of clinical medicine (79). Featuring lighter inclusion criteria, more varied treatment settings, "softer" endpoints, and the allowance of concurrent treatments, effectiveness studies produce less reliable results due to their greater statistical noise. (These studies have lower front-end rigor but higher back-end rigor.) The Institute of Medicine's Committee on CAM helpfully distinguishes the two kinds of studies in teleological terms: "Efficacy refers to what a treatment *can* do under ideal circumstances; effectiveness refers to what a treatment *does* do in routine daily use" (Committee 104; original emphasis).

CAM practices do not fit well within an efficacy model. Practices such as traditional Chinese medicine and chiropractic are much more amenable to effectiveness studies because such studies can better accommodate the sorts of patients, symptoms, treatments, and outcomes typical of their patient populations. CAM users tend to use multiple modalities concurrently, including biomedical ones, so ethical questions would arise in an efficacy study, since that model would restrict participants' ability to combine therapies in order to determine causality of treatment effects. Likewise, endpoints of CAM studies usually need to be softer (i.e., more subjective, usually patient-reported) than those of efficacy studies because patients typically seek CAM for chronic, intractable conditions, such as those lacking clear prognoses and/or treatment, and those associated with hard-to-measure symptoms such as pain and fatigue.

Critics of research on CAM both within the *JAMA-Archives* theme issues and beyond typically hold up efficacy, not effectiveness, as the criterion by which CAM should be evaluated, even though much biomedical research is effectiveness-based (and still more is based on observational studies, which are neither randomized nor controlled).[16] Not surprisingly, however, even when efficacy studies of CAM are available, such as Cardini and Weixin's and Shlay et al.'s acupuncture trials, their methods tend to be subjected to greater scrutiny than are their biomedical counterparts (Borgerson; Morreim). Certainly, given the studies' complex design challenges, it seems only fair to exercise some caution when evaluating their results. However, much of the skepticism about CAM's potential efficacy that is expressed both within the *JAMA-Archives* theme issues (e.g., Delbanco; Happle; Smolle, Prause, and Kerl) and in my interviews with researchers Clarke and Fournier and physician-clinician McDonald stems not from doubt about the study's design but from doubt about the study intervention itself.

Fournier, for example, struggled to articulate his response to Cardini and Weixin's positive result—75 percent of breech fetuses in the intervention group were head-first at 35 weeks' gestation vs. 48 percent of those in the control group. As he read through the study's results section, he paused for more than thirty seconds, silently scanning the text. He explained, flipping back and forth through the article, "Just trying to see if it's biased in some way. I don't know if I'm missing something." He continued to talk himself through the methods and results, frequently pausing and restarting as he tried to make sense of the evidence of effect in the study's intervention group, which he described, with a laugh, as "pretty high." When I asked whether he would be as curious about the study's design if the result were negative, he admitted, "I might not be as critical, to be quite frank."

Prior to reaching this section in the Cardini and Weixin study, Fournier had been reasonably satisfied with its methods and its ability to demonstrate whether moxibustion had an effect on breech pregnancies. While reading through the results, however, he invoked a stricter set of criteria for proof of efficacy. In admitting that he would likely be less scrupulous with a negative finding, Fournier reveals the kind of double-standard that Morreim notes is characteristic of most biomedical research on CAM, one that is evinced throughout the *JAMA-Archives* theme issues (e.g., Delbanco; Happle; Smolle, Prause, and Kerl). As this example shows, although efficacy is a shared multi-disciplinary concept that enables research on CAM (i.e., it is a boundary object), it can also be invoked in a more restricted sense by some participants to reshape issues into a framework more amenable with their own perspective.[17]

In mainstream drug trials, there is also a more insidious side to the notion of efficacy that can illustrate how its elasticity can be manipulated in debates about CAM to distort scientific practices and advance particular argumentative aims. Measures employed in biomedical research to ensure objectivity, for instance, may be actively manipulated to produce desired results. In such circumstances, *efficacy* takes on new meaning because it comes to mean whatever the triallists engineer it to mean. Former *New England Journal of Medicine* editor Marcia Angell's incisive exposé of pharmaceutical research and marketing is emblematic of the new culture of criticism surrounding medical research. In the book, she describes the manifold ways that drug companies manipulate trial design and results to skew evidence in their favor. For example, researchers may alter inclusion criteria to include younger participants in studies of interventions designed for elderly patients in order to "engineer out" untoward side effects, since younger participants tend to experience fewer. Similarly, studies can manipulate dosing regimens to "engineer up" the efficacy of the study drug in head-to-head trials (i.e., drug-against-drug, rather than drug-against-placebo). One such strategy is to administer the comparator treatment, usually one with established efficacy, at half the normal effective dose or in a nonstandard format (e.g., tablet form rather than injected). As the chief scientific officer of one research facility remarked to anthropologist Adriana Petryna, of such strategies of dosage manipulation, "That is the big game of clinical trials" (27; see also Angell 107–09; Dumit, *Drugs*). These strategies exploit the concept of efficacy to favor a drug company's own products, especially in cases where the study drug is no more effective than competitor interventions. By halving the dose of a competitor product, one's own product looks all the more effective by comparison.

More extreme still, in terms of altering evidence of efficacy in biomedicine, is when unfavorable research results are suppressed. This occurs when companies sponsoring research try to control the impact of studies with negative results by effectively burying them, or by presenting only partial evidence that shows a positive effect, or by spinning negative results to highlight, for example, subpopulations of the trial for which the drug did work (Angell 109–11). For example, when an AIDS "therapeutic vaccine," Remune, proved ineffective, the sponsoring company Immune Response Corporation attempted to muzzle university-based researchers from disseminating the results, since those results would imperil its product (Angell).

Still more damning is the landmark case of the Apotex trial of deferiprone, an iron-chelation agent for the inherited blood disorder thalassemia. When Nancy Olivieri, the University of Toronto-based researcher who was investigating the drug at the Toronto Hospital for Sick Children, became concerned in 1995 about the drug's effectiveness and potential toxicity, she brought her concerns to both the sponsoring company, Apotex, and the hospital research ethics board (REB) overseeing the research. Under the REB's orders, Olivieri requested that informed consent forms be altered to disclose potential risks to participants but the company refused. Citing a confidentiality agreement she had signed with the company at the start of the research trials, the company expressly forbade her from communicating her concerns to participants or other researchers. Olivieri refused to bend to Apotex's will and her research contract was terminated, leading to several years of protracted institutional and bureaucratic wrangling that saw Olivieri temporarily lose her job (Viens and Savulescu). In 1998, Olivieri and colleagues published their findings in the *New England Journal of Medicine*; the drug was eventually approved for use in the United States but has not yet been approved in Canada.

To be sure, these strategies for manipulating evidence of efficacy in drug trials are not carried out in the name of boundary work: as a growing mass of studies illustrate, such manipulation results directly from industry involvement in research.[18] (If the companies are paying for the studies, the thinking seems to go, then they should have a say in what sorts of results they produce.) What is important here is that if we think of efficacy as a boundary object with rhetorical mobility, then this highly specialized, if frequently deceptive, notion of "proving" health interventions can help to demonstrate how ephemeral a concept efficacy can be. Dismissals of CAM that hinge on the idea of efficacy thus seem to be motivated at least in part by a demarcation exigence, to use Wilson and Herndl's phrase, because those dismissals use a concept that is *flexible* within biomedicine to draw *inflexible* boundary lines around it. That is, while "efficacy" has a range of meanings in biomedicine, some softer than others, that range is considerably less elastic at the edges of biomedicine. The criteria for determining whether or not an intervention "works" seem to be narrower, and firmer, for evaluations of CAM than they are for biomedicine.

Tom Delbanco's damnation of CAM as a glorified placebo in the *JAMA* theme issue is a good case in point. Although he laments that "the public should not stand for spending tax revenues on studies not worth doing," he expresses relief that such studies will at least "shatter claims for activity beyond placebo" (1561). The prospect of such an outcome confirming placebo effects bothered neither Connolly nor Yao, the traditional Chinese medical practitioners that I interviewed, because, as Connolly explained, there "is no such thing" as a placebo effect in traditional Chinese medicine. Body and mind are considered together as a whole so, in the end, it does not matter whether effects of treatment occur in patients' physical meridians or in their spirit. Indeed, Yao claimed this latter "spirit" effect as an integral aspect of his practice:

> I could just touch you, right, and you would think, "Oh the needle is in now." That, we call [a] "Positive Psychological Effect." We didn't do anything, actually, only your psychology will produce the results. And MDs and scientists have criticized us very often about this practice. They say, "Oh TCM-acupuncture is psychology." Well, psychology is good. [*Laughs.*] We can produce thirty percent results [that way], according to one [study]. Thirty percent.

In the framework of evidence-based medicine, this model of practice would likely constitute fraud, and even the most open-minded medical doctor or researcher might worry about its ethics. However, Yao's attitude toward patient psychology is not anomalous in complementary and alternative medicine, and this is one of the leading charges against CAM practitioners, that their "healing" consists not in their therapies but in their clinical dispositions and their invocation of placebo effects. Since biomedical studies of CAM practices are often difficult to blind and control, one question often remains about them: If patients experienced improvement, was it due to actual physiological effects or just placebo effects? The criteria adopted in answering this question directly inform the ways in which efficacy can be invoked as a rhetorical boundary object.

The idea of the placebo effect is based on an additive model. Ted Kaptchuk, trained in traditional Chinese medicine and now the director of the Harvard Program in Placebo Studies and the Therapeutic Encounter, notes that since all arms of a study are expected to "receive equal and independent amounts" of this effect, the belief is that "one could simply subtract the amount of placebo effect to determine the presence (or absence) of specific drug effect" ("Powerful" 1724). However, this model does not allow for what he calls a "differential" placebo effect among arms, where participants receiving different treatments may experience different kinds or amounts of placebo effects, which is a very real possibility in CAM research because it is so difficult to create sham interventions that are both realistic and definitely inert.

Consider, for instance, the uneven distribution of placebo in the Cardini and Weixin trial: the intervention group received special training at the hospital, brought home with them tangible objects for treatment (the *moxa* rolls, made of Artemisia leaves), and spent thirty minutes of each day of the study in close physical proximity to a loved one administering the therapy, while control group received no treatment at all, aside from standard maternity care. To mitigate the differences between treatment arms, Cardini and Weixin could have used a different material in the moxa rolls or placed the rolls in a location other than the selected acupoint, but each of these approaches could have introduced new, unintended treatment effects that would complicate assessment of the trial intervention. The control acupoints in the Shlay study pose similar problems: because both intervention and control needles were actually inserted into the skin, we cannot know for sure whether neither SAR nor placebo had effects or both SAR and placebo had effects, and if so, the weighted effects of each.

Depending on where one sits in the boundary zone between biomedicine and CAM, placebo controls take on different levels of importance in determining an intervention's efficacy. For skeptics such as Delbanco, the problems of identifying appropriate placebo controls in CAM can be traced to defects in the practices themselves—his own take is that they cannot be tested against placebos because they *are* placebos. For those with a more moderate view of CAM, however, placebo controls play a less clear role in the evaluation of efficacy because, although they are central to RCT design, they are not nearly the safeguard against bias that the literature on evidence-based medicine would have one believe. For one, placebos can also be manipulated to rig clinical trials and skew their results. The notion of "targeted efficacy" in antidepressant trials (Lakoff 65), for instance, allows researchers to seek not the right drug for patients but "the right patients for the drug." In such cases, triallists aim to find participants who readily "pick up the signal" of the study drug rather than test it in a wider participant population (65). Furthermore, although many critics of CAM research decry studies that do not use what they believe to be adequate placebo controls, use of placebos can often be unethical, particularly when alternatives with known or suspected efficacy are available. (See, e.g., Maguire on placebo use in HIV research.) Given that patients often seek CAM for chronic pain (as in the Shlay study), the possibility that half the trial population might be given nothing at all could be ethically troubling.[19] The relative weight that commentators assign to the use placebo controls in debates about CAM seems to inform their assessment of a given practice's efficacy.

What these examples show is that we can think of the meaning of boundary objects—in this case, the notion of efficacy—as having a certain degree of mobility for only some of the actors involved. My argument here builds on Wilson and Herndl's examination of how cooperation among members of a multidisciplinary work group at the Los Alamos National Laboratory is facilitated by what they call knowledge maps, visual representations of team members' areas of expertise, functions, and interrelations within the work group. These knowledge maps served in the group as boundary objects, enabling team members to speak to one another across disciplinary (and conceptual) lines. Wilson and Herndl recast Star and Griesemer's concept of the boundary object into a rhetorical framework by showing how knowledge maps produce what Peter Galison calls a "trading zone," a temporary site for the "*local* coordination" of distinct groups with "vast *global* differences" (Galison 783; emphasis in original). The examples I have cited in this section do not fit exactly within Wilson and Herndl's model, however: while cooperation is the order of the day in biomedical CAM research, there are specific, if limited, instances wherein biomedical actors can reshape *efficacy* as a boundary object to alter favorably the terms of the debate.

I would argue, then, that there is overlap between the boundary object trading zone, a site of interdisciplinary collaboration, and what Michael Gorman calls the "élite" trading zone. In an élite trading zone, Gorman argues, "a group of experts use their specialized knowledge to dictate how a sociotechnical system will function. The expertise of such an élite is black-boxed for other participants in the network" (933). This is a zone in which no meaningful trade in expertise takes place. In CAM research, access to the notion of efficacy appears to be partially black-boxed to some of the participants some of the time, which allows other, more powerful participants to control, if temporarily, what it means to say a given health practice works. The rhetorical mobility of efficacy as a boundary object has important implications for both CAM-related research and medicine more generally: it shapes what we know about health interventions and how we know it. The study of efficacy from a rhetorical perspective can thus offer important insight when we ask, as Taubes did, "Do we really know what makes us healthy?"

∗

Around the same time that the randomized controlled trial began its ascent as the premiere means of producing evidence on which health interventions work and which do not, rhetorical scholar Donald C. Bryant famously defined rhetoric as the "art of adjusting ideas to people and people to ideas" (420). While these two events occurred in different arenas, Bryant's notion of "adjusting" people and ideas to one another resonates with the substance of this chapter because the randomized controlled trial is, among other things, a thoroughly rhetorical concept. In biomedical boundary work, the RCT can be invoked variously to sponsor identification or division among stakeholders in the research, but only certain ideas and certain people need to be "adjusted": those with fewer rhetorical resources. Note, for example, Margolin, Avants, and Kleber's conclusion in their *JAMA* editorial that "controlled evaluation of [CAM] may require its practitioners to undertake a fundamental conceptual shift from a view of patients as requiring individualized treatment . . . to one in which trial participants are regarded as members of an equivalence class, defined by the diagnosis, who all will be given a standard prescribed treatment" (1627). Biomedicine is not asked here to undergo a "conceptual shift" because it provides the very context of the debate—it sets the terms and conditions its outcome.

Connolly, the traditional Chinese medicine practitioner I interviewed for this book, recognized this need for a conceptual shift in his own practice, noting the importance of being able to move fluidly between Eastern and Western concepts of health and illness: "We have to [be able to switch]. The Western . . . medical community will not talk our language ever, so if we don't talk to them, it's like two people in different languages trying to communicate and get along. It doesn't work very well." Of course, proponents of CAM may not all willingly go along with the idea of adjusting their basic premises and their principles of practice to the biomedical model. However, should they wish to attain legitimacy within the biomedical community, it seems likely that they will have to continue to "adjust" themselves to biomedicine because the boundary dispute is partly fixed, and not in their favor.

As this chapter has argued, method functions in the *JAMA-Archives* theme issues as a rhetorical topos that can be invoked in arguments about complementary and alternative medicine to draw professional and epistemic boundary lines. However, this argument is complicated by the complicated position that methodology in turn holds in biomedicine: although the randomized controlled trial is revered as medicine's primary source of "best evidence," its *actual* evidence-producing ability is less assured. As philosopher of science Nancy Cartwright notes in her assessment of the RCT:

> There is no gold standard; no universally best method. Gold standard methods are whatever methods will provide (a) the information you need, (b) reliably, (c) from what you can do and from what you can know on the occasion. Often randomized controlled trials (RCTs) are very bad at this and other methods very good. What method best provides the information you want reliably will differ from case to case, depending primarily on what you already know or can come to know. (11)

Cartwright's conclusion is compatible with Sackett and colleagues' own view, in their treatise on evidence-based medicine, that although RCT-derived evidence is the most reliable form of evidence, it is certainly not the only valid form. In circumstances where RCT evidence is not available for a given question, Sackett et al. assert simply that "we must follow the trail to the next best external evidence and work from there" (72). In the medical literature on CAM, however, that "trail" of evidence often leads right back to the RCT, a circularity that can be traced to the evidence-based movement and the demarcation exigence that it precipitates. In the context of biomedical-CAM boundary work, then, *method* can be strategically invoked, eulogistically or dyslogistically, depending on a given commentator's perspective.

Studying how the arguments from method advanced in the *JAMA-Archives* theme issues do not match up with the methods adopted in everyday medical research can magnify problems that have always been central in biomedicine but largely unarticulated. That is, these studies on complementary and alternative medicine can offer clearer ways of seeing how certain forms of evidence can be marshaled rhetorically to draw professional and epistemic boundary lines.

Of course, methodological rigor is the centerpiece of medical research and studies cannot be designed haphazardly. However, since genres such as RCT reports are community-based—they represent communally held values about what counts as proper evidence—trials of CAM can be illuminating because those communal values do not quite hold. CAM practices thrive outside of the biomedical sphere and, while the major ones (such as acupuncture and chiropractic) have increasingly come to work in concert with biomedicine, their practitioners remain strangers in the community of medical scientists. The strangeness of CAM interventions within biomedical borders can bring into relief biomedicine's own idealized model of research, manifest in the framework of evidence-based medicine, wherein the best evidence for a particular health intervention seems to have little to do with patients themselves; this is the subject of the next chapter.

Precincts of Care in CAM Research

In considering this book's guiding question—*How does the notion of evidence determine the boundaries of biomedicine, from expert to public contexts?*—the previous chapters have examined the performance of boundary work upstream in the realm of medical research on complementary and alternative medicine (CAM). Those chapters analyzed the 1998 CAM-themed issues of the *Journal of the American Medical Association* and its associated *Archives* journals to show how the notion of evidence defines and circumscribes the limits of acceptable knowledge, how medical researchers and practitioners define and categorize the practices that comprise CAM, and how researchers design and interpret clinical studies of CAM interventions. The present chapter moves further downstream to examine how the *JAMA-Archives* theme issues configure biomedical boundaries within contexts of care. Scientific research on CAM traverses boundaries among models of medical practice that can be illuminated by studying how the journals configure practitioner-patient interaction, the most unambiguously rhetorical element of clinical medicine.

Much of the everyday practice of medicine hinges on rhetorical engagement: patients must persuade physicians that they are injured or ill and in need of diagnosis and treatment, particularly in cases where patients do not have observable symptoms such as visible wounds, palpable tumors, or measurable fevers; physicians must persuade patients to submit to diagnostic tests, follow courses of treatment, and seek consultations with specialists. Increasingly, physicians are tasked with persuading worried patients that they do not require treatment even despite their feeling ill. The language that practitioners and patients use in contexts of care is also persuasive, even if it is not intended to be so. For example, metaphors of war that are commonly used in cancer care and end-of-life care (e.g., "you're a fighter"; "she lost her battle") negatively affect patient outcomes because they frame cancer and dying as competitive struggles that involve opponents and winners and losers.[1] How practitioners and patients work on, with, and against one another in clinical settings can importantly shape health outcomes. Even incidental forms of interaction in the clinic, such as small talk, eye contact, and touching, can affect whether and how patients respond to care.

The question of how to evaluate health interventions in which the clinical encounter may itself have therapeutic value has increasingly been fore-grounded as health research agendas have adopted more encompassing views of health and illness. In Canada, for example, the replacement in 2000 of the federal Medical Research Council with the Canadian Institutes of Health Research recognized that advances in biomedicine are a key factor, but not the only factor, in improving the overall health of Canadians.[2] This movement toward a broader focus in health research stems in large part from rising incidence of chronic, functional conditions, such as pain, fatigue, impaired cognitive function, and intestinal discomfort—conditions for which conventional medicine is often not able to offer much relief. Patients with such conditions seem to benefit, especially, from care that involves an interpersonal dimension (Barry et al.; Wagner et al.). However, health interventions that depend on interaction among practitioners and patients do not fit easily in an evidence-based framework because they are difficult to investigate through biomedicine's gold-standard methodology, the randomized controlled trial (RCT). RCTs aim to isolate interventions from their contexts of delivery through randomization, double-blinding, and placebo controls, but many interventions are embedded within those contexts and so are difficult to isolate and test. This is true not only of many CAM practices but also of conventional medicine, in areas such as clinical care, nursing, and hospital units *qua* units. Such interventions are not easily randomized, blinded, or controlled because they comprise multiple, contingent, and interactive effects that cannot be isolated the way that a single drug's effects can be.

As the previous chapter illustrates, in debates about CAM, questions of research methodology can be invoked to shift boundaries of what counts as safe and effective health care and what does not. The present chapter extends that claim to argue that the configuration of practitioner-patient interaction in research contexts is also persuasive: interaction, and ideas about interaction, can persuade us toward different views on the conduct of biomedical research on CAM and on the place of patients within health care contexts more generally. In the sections that follow, I argue that biomedical boundaries are negotiated in part through the ways that research accounts for practice, particularly because, within evidence-based medicine, the ability of individual interventions to integrate research-derived evidence into practice can persuade us to value those interventions above others not so amenable to experimental research.

Firenzuoli and Gori capture part of this tension between research and practice in a letter they submitted to the *British Medical Journal* in response to Sackett et al.'s influential 1996 article on evidence-based medicine (EBM): "While clinicians are exhorted to use up to date research evidence to give patients the best possible care, actually doing so in individual patients is difficult: at the heart of clinical medicine is an unresolved conflict between the essentially case based nature of clinical practice and the mainly population based nature of the research evidence." The tension that I want to illuminate in this chapter lies even deeper than Firenzuoli and Gori's focus on clinical implementation, the unidirectional application of evidence to patient care. Rather than examine whether and how research figures into clinical practice, as they do, I turn things around to examine whether and how practice figures into research. How are interventions that depend significantly on practitioner-patient interaction tested experimentally, and what is gained and lost in the process for health care delivery, patient care, and medical-professional boundary work?

Interventions with diverse and indeterminate interactive effects have been variously categorized in the medical literature as "complex" (Blackwood), "complex composite" (van Weel and Knottnerus), "socially complex" (Wolff), and "sentient" (Lindsay). While these designations vary in their specificity, they all align substantially with the UK Medical Research Council description: "Complex interventions in health care, whether therapeutic or preventative, comprise a number of separate elements which seem essential to the proper functioning of the intervention although the 'active ingredient' of the intervention that is effective is difficult to specify" (1). The descriptive limits of such interventions are blurry even in this formal definition, but the council offers a useful heuristic: "The greater the difficulty in defining precisely what, exactly, are the 'active ingredients' of an intervention and how they relate to each other, the greater the likelihood that you are dealing with a complex intervention" (1).

Professionalized CAM modalities such as acupuncture and chiropractic fit well within the rubric of socially complex interventions because they consist of what health services researchers Paterson and Dieppe call "complex packages of care" (1204; see also MacPherson, Thorpe, and Thomas; Mason, Tovey, and Long). Chiropractic, for instance, involves a multifaceted approach, no part of which is alone sufficient to care, including patient education, psychosocial counsel, sustained physical contact, spinal adjustment, and patient self-care (Oths, "Communication," "Unintended Therapy"). However, while CAM practices align well with biomedical interventions that are socially complex (such as nursing), they remain strange enough within a mainstream medical context that their efficacy is often strongly suspect and skeptics often dismiss evidence of efficacy in CAM as the product of placebo effects rather than of any real physiological effect. Recall, for example, Tom Delbanco's dismissal of CAM discussed in the previous chapter: linking CAM's apparent efficacy to interactive effects such as increased attention to patients' quality of life and needs for comfort, he confidently asserts in the *JAMA* theme issue that "academic medicine will soon shatter claims for activity [in CAM] beyond placebo" (1561).

Biomedical research on CAM practices such as acupuncture and chiropractic tends to treat those practices' characteristically higher levels of individualized care and practitioner-patient interaction as a potential contaminant, as something to be controlled for through innovative design. In the Shlay study from the previous chapter, for example, the researchers adopted a standardized acupuncture protocol to treat HIV-related nerve damage, but in actual practice, treatment would depend on individualized assessment and discussion between practitioner and patient. By controlling for interactive effects by eliminating those elements of individualization, research on CAM consequently sponsors a model of health care at odds with both the rhetorical conditions governing clinical practice and the guiding philosophies of CAM practices that depend on talk, touch, and whole-person care.

In this chapter, I follow the thread of practitioner-patient interaction through the varied theoretical geographies of research on CAM to frame some of biomedicine's larger epistemic processes in more concrete terms. This process of reframing biomedical research on CAM within the context of practice, vis-à-vis practitioner-patient interaction, can ultimately reveal the theoretical terrain of medicine itself. The chapter begins by situating socially complex interventions in the context of contemporary theoretical models of medical practice. The second section examines rhetorical interaction as a potential contaminant in biomedical research on CAM, while the third reflects, in particular, on what CAM trials can tell us about what are usually thought of as placebo effects, which have strong links to practitioner-patient interaction. The fourth section considers patient agency and the limits of patient choice in clinical consultations, both mainstream and alternative. The fifth section further examines patient agency by focusing on discourses surrounding dietary supplements and the possibility that individuals use supplements in part to gain a greater sense of control over their own health.

The awkward fit between medical research and the practice it is ostensibly meant to inform illuminates some of the disabling assumptions behind evidence-based medicine. It also draws attention to the ways in which increasingly expansive views of health and illness can both humanize health care delivery *and* bolster further medicalization of ordinary human life. As an extreme case within the wider domain of research on socially complex interventions, studies of complementary and alternative medicine can amplify potential conflicts at the heart of medical research more generally. For example, attempts in CAM studies to control for biases and therapeutic effects arising from practitioner-patient interaction can be seen, more globally, as probes into the relationship in mainstream medicine between health care providers and patients. These probes illuminate the interactional dimensions of some of biomedicine's most intractable problems, such as patient compliance/concordance and overdependence on pharmaceuticals. The chapter closes with some reflection on these issues.

Models of Clinical Practice

The move in scholarship on health beyond a model of disease as essentially organic, rooted in biological pathology, has unfolded unevenly, shaped by tensions between evidence-based medicine and patient-centered care, two multidimensional approaches to medicine that have gained currency in recent decades. While patient-centered care is a model of practice predicated on involving patients and their families more directly in their own care, evidence-based medicine provides a justification for clinical decision-making—it is a model not *of* professional practice but rather *governing* professional practice. Both evidence-based medicine and patient-centered care play a significant role in the testing of socially complex interventions, including CAM practices such as traditional Chinese medicine and chiropractic.

The widespread impulse to test socially complex interventions through randomized controlled trials, despite their poor fit with the methodology, derives from emergent trends toward risk management and accountability within the context of evidence-based medicine. This shift in turn sponsors the expansion of experimental methods into areas previously tested only by other means (e.g., observation). As evidence-based medicine increasingly privileged data derived from randomized controlled trials, other methodologies began to fall short by comparison; through that process, advocates of evidence-based medicine consequently emphasized results derived from hard endpoints—"death, disease, and demography" (Committee 105)—over softer endpoints identified by subjective measures such as pain scales and patient diaries. The problem for socially complex interventions, not only in CAM but also within biomedicine, is that their effects are generally not measurable through quantitative means.

This quantitative bent in health research has contributed to the marginalization of practices even in mainstream biomedicine that are not directly amenable to experimental methods. As nursing scholar Bronagh Blackwood notes, "A clear definition, the ability to control outside factors and standardization of the intervention are the cornerstones of the RCT" (612); socially complex interventions fail on all three counts and more. The most significant problems that the RCT format poses for these interventions include defining the parameters of the intervention (Lindsay; Medical Research Council), standardizing and controlling it (Wolff), and randomizing trial participants either to receive it or not (van Weel and Knottnerus).

The marginalization of interaction-dependent interventions has led, in part, to the development of patient-centered care. It is a bit strange to think of patient-centered care as merely a model of practice, since everything in medicine is ostensibly done in the name of the patient, but as rhetorician Charles Anderson has observed, although the patient is "the center of the medical event," he or she, as a person, tends to be taken as "merely attached to the machine delivered up for repair" (6). Compounding this limited view of the patient as a machine is a limited view in contemporary biomedicine of the patient as an interlocutor. Clinical encounters can frequently be rhetorically disabling for patients because they occur within well-established hierarchies under circumstances generally beyond the patient's control (Ong et al. 903). In such a dynamic, anthropologist Christine Barry and colleagues explain, "The voice of medicine has doctors maintaining control within a power imbalance. As a result the coherent and meaningful accounts of patients are suppressed," resulting in "disruption and fragmentation of communication" (Barry et al. 489).

Empirical research illustrates just how disrupted and fragmented biomedical care can be: one study of doctor-patient communication in the late 1980s found, for example, that more than two-thirds of physicians interrupted their patients' opening statements within eighteen seconds (Frankel and Beckman 88), while another study, from the mid 1990s, found that doctors contributed at least 60 percent of clinical talk (Ong et al. 906). This asymmetrical discursive environment can impede a patient's sense of agency in her own health care in the clinical setting. Note, for example, the tenor of these current popular book titles: *How to Talk to Your Doctor: Getting the Answers and Care You Need* (Agnew); *What Your Doctor Really Thinks: Diagnosing the Doctor-Patient Relationship* (Blumer; emphasis in original); *Patient Beware! Dealing*

With Doctors and Other Medical Dilemmas (Carver). The wide availability of these and similar self-help handbooks—even the American Medical Association has produced one (Perry)—signals that something has gone awry in doctor-patient communication.

Patient-centered care is predicated on the idea that we need to offset the technoscientific, doctor-oriented discourse that pervades much of medicine today, to restore the whole patient, as an individual agent, to the medical encounter by providing "care that is concordant with the patient's values, needs and preferences, and that allows patients to provide input and participate actively in decisions regarding their health and health care" (Epstein et al. 1516).[3] For many critics and researchers, communication, broadly conceived, is "the royal pathway to patient-centered care" (Bensing 23). Note, for instance, this account in Siegfried Meryn's 1998 editorial in the *British Medical Journal*:

> Most complaints by patients and the public about doctors deal with problems of communication not with clinical competency. The commonest complaint is that doctors do not listen to them. Patients want more and better information about their problem and the outcome, more openness about the side effects of treatment, relief of pain and emotional distress, and advice on what they can do for themselves. (1922)

Extensive scholarship on doctor-patient interaction has demonstrated that communication is integral to successful medical encounters. Patient outcomes have been positively correlated with, for example, longer clinical encounters, more detailed history-taking, and increased psychosocial talk, eye contact, and touching; outcomes have been negatively correlated with high levels of biomedical questioning, directive behavior, and interruptions (see, e.g., Beck, Daughtridge, and Sloane; Mishler; Stewart and Roter).

In complementary and alternative medicine, communication is central to most clinical encounters, and many practitioners consciously cultivate their communicative skills in both their initial training and their ongoing education. Tao Liu notes of acupuncture, for example, that the "treatment session is characterized, except for needle insertion itself, by the elaborate and comprehensive communication between the acupuncturist and the patient" (4). Similarly, MacPherson, Thorpe, and Thomas characterize acupuncture as fundamentally patient-centered, "based on a partnership model of interaction between practitioner and patient" nurtured by "establishing rapport with patients, active listening, and utilizing explanatory models" based on Chinese medical philosophy to create a common theoretical understanding of the patient's condition and treatment (878). Although the quantity of talk in acupuncture practice may not always be high, the practitioner-patient relationship is still central to treatment, supported for example through nonverbal actions such as touching the patient's body and listening to its sounds, and through its central focus on holism (Ho and Bylund 513).

CAM practitioners' explicit attention to communication may contribute significantly to CAM's growing popularity as prevalence of chronic illness rises. Anthropologist Kathryn Oths explains, for example, that "Chiropractors are in demand because they supply what is often absent from overly logical and rational modern medicine—more social, psychological, and physical interaction, more listening, empathy, support, reassurance, and touching" ("Unintended" 88; see also Vincent and Furnham 37). Although practices such as traditional Chinese medicine and chiropractic may not ultimately be as patient-centered as their proponents suggest, the priority they accord to interaction between practitioners and patients nevertheless stands in sharp contrast to that of biomedicine.

The patient-centered care model is not without criticism, particularly regarding the feasibility of implementing such a potentially time-consuming approach to practice in an age of managed care and fee-for-service programs. However, in the context of evidence-based medicine, patient-centered care offers an important corrective to the valorization of trial evidence—a valorization that physicians Feinstein and Horwitz worry will "produce inappropriate guidelines or doctrinaire dogmas for clinical practice," wherein doctors "may often be diverted from the bedside to the library or computer terminal" (533). Although it turns out that the patient-centered model does not always translate well into actual medical practice, the premium that the model places on understanding the social complexities of care demonstrates that, even in an evidence-based framework, interaction between practitioners and patients may have substantial, and possibly measurable, effects on patient outcomes.

Regulating Rhetorical Interaction

Practitioner-patient interaction is difficult to measure empirically in any medical model, mainstream or alternative, so it is difficult to develop an evidence base on matters of the interaction and its effect on treatment. However, given that disputes over the validity of CAM practices generally hinge on whether or not their efficacy has been demonstrated in randomized controlled trials, the difficulty of generating evidence on interactive effects in CAM elicits questions in the context of boundary work that are more than procedural (e.g., "How can one measure the effects of clinical interaction in an RCT?"). This difficulty of generating evidence also elicits epistemological questions that can ultimately cast the validity of the CAM practice itself into doubt (e.g., "By what biological mechanism, if any, does the intervention actually work?"; "Is the effect anything more than placebo?") Following on these epistemological questions, I argue in this section that trials of acupuncture and chiropractic published in the *JAMA-Archives* theme issues document researchers' attempts to regulate rhetorical interaction between practitioners and patients—all of the ways in which they act on and with one another, consciously and not—in order to produce legitimate evidence on the interventions' safety and efficacy.

The studies I examine here include those analyzed in the previous chapter, Cardini and Weixin's trial of moxibustion (the burning of herb rolls on acupuncture points) for breech pregnancies and Shlay et al.'s trial of standardized acupuncture for HIV-related neuropathy, as well as Bove and Nilsson's trial of chiropractic adjustment for the treatment of tension headache. By positing practitioner-patient interaction as a contaminant, a potentially confounding variable, these clinical trials propose models of practice that conflict with what we know about why patients seek alternative practitioners (Astin) and about the importance of practitioner-patient communication to patient outcomes (Beck, Daughtridge, and Sloane).

Among the primary reasons that patients give for seeking CAM are that they report receiving greater interpersonal attention and that they find such practices more congruent with their own attitudes toward health and illness. Patients with chronic, functional symptoms, who make up the majority of CAM users, particularly value the attention given in CAM not only to their diseases but, more importantly, to their illness experiences. Busby notes, for example, that people who feel their illness experiences have been "distort[ed]" within a medical lexicon tend to find CAM practices "more congruent with their experience of their own bodies, and lifeworlds" (qtd. in Barry et al. 489). In CAM, Busby argues, the patient's physiological condition generally does not take precedence as it does in mainstream medicine but is, instead, deliberately situated within the larger context of the patient's "lifeworld."[4]

Practitioner-patient communication lies at the center of most discussions of why patients choose CAM. For instance, in the editorial materials from *JAMA* and the *Archives* that I discussed in the previous chapter, commentators such as Jonas, Koo and Arain, and O'Sullivan, Lipper, and Lerner identify biomedicine's shortcomings in clinical interaction as a driving force behind the popularity of CAM. More recent commentaries corroborate this view as well. For example, health sociologist Merrijoy Kelner cites CAM's interactivity as its key selling point, arguing that CAM practitioners are more empathetic and collaborative than mainstream physicians, and that they make the therapeutic relationship a priority, fostering strong practitioner-patient rapport. Pappas and Perlman similarly cite longer appointments, more detailed explanation of illness and treatment, greater continuity of care, and "attention to personality and personal experience" as major attractions of CAM (3), particularly because patient satisfaction in CAM "often is not dependent on an improvement in the presenting complaint" (3).

For patients with chronic conditions, the trick seems less to be to improve the chronic symptoms themselves than to improve patients' experience of those symptoms. A shift in the care of chronic illness from quantitative assessment (lab tests, x-rays, scans) to qualitative assessment (questionnaires, interviews, diaries) makes sense because the conditions are typically ongoing. Ultimately, the appeal of CAM practices for such patients may be that the practices provide patients "a participatory experience of empowerment, authenticity, and enlarged self-identity when illness threatens [patients'] sense of intactness and connection to the world" (Kaptchuk and Eisenberg, "Persuasive Appeal" 1061).

In a biomedical framework, the kind of patient-centeredness found in CAM comes at the expense of evidence: the evidence base of practices such as acupuncture and chiropractic relies primarily on theory and anecdote, evidence not nearly sufficient to justify their use within an evidence-based framework. (Note the widely circulated aphorism in EBM that the plural of "anecdote" is not "data.") Evidence-based approaches to CAM reframe those practices within a biomedical terminology. In acupuncture for pain relief, for example, traditional Chinese medical theories of energy flow and blockage are replaced by biochemical and genetic mechanisms, such as the release of "ß-endorphin, an endogenous opioid with high affinity for the μ-receptor . . . into the blood from the hypothalamus via the anterior pituitary" (Stener-Victorin et al. 1943) and "gene expression of peptides for central pain control" (Ulett 1271). The Shlay et al. study of acupuncture for HIV-related nerve damage is a good case in point: it carefully details the protocol for acupuncture needle insertion and manipulation but not its theoretical basis, only hinting in the article's conclusion that its mechanism is likely biochemical: "the release of endogenous opioids or activation of other brain and spinal cord pathways that reduce pain" (1594). In the contest for scientific legitimacy, this shift away from traditional Chinese meridian theory makes sense if researchers want to identify a biomedically plausible mechanism for acupuncture's effect.

The movement away from traditional acupuncture theory, a strategy long adopted in the *American Journal of Chinese Medicine*, reflects the researchers' anxiety in the *JAMA-Archives* to strengthen their studies' ties to biomedicine by reframing the practice into a more amenable framework. In this process

of reframing, however, biomedical acupuncture studies often end up eliminating the very qualities that draw patients to acupuncture in the first place.
For example, in a letter published in *JAMA* in 1999 in response to the Shlay
et al. study, George Ulett reports of physicians with conventional MD degrees
learning to perform acupuncture, divorced entirely from traditional Chinese
medical theory. Ulett praises this new, physician-applied acupuncture as a
sign of progress, learned in only a few hours of training rather than the 1,500
hours of training he cites as recommended for traditional acupuncturists. For
some patients, physician-based acupuncture may provide just the relief they
need. However, for patients seeking a holistic practice that offers individualized treatment within a therapeutic relationship, physician-based acupuncture
may not provide the care they wish to have because, in that model, needling is
abstracted from the range of interventions typically provided concurrently in
traditional Chinese medicine (herbal remedies, cupping, moxibustion, massage, and lifestyle modifications such as dietary changes and exercise) and re-
contextualized within a biomedical framework. In such a case, we might think
of the perspectives of doctors and patients as fundamentally misaligned.

The distance between the perspectives of doctors and patients can usefully be captured by Kenneth Burke's well-known observation that language is
not only a reflection of reality but also a selection and deflection of reality. As
Burke says, "we can't say anything without the use of terms; whatever terms we
use, they necessarily constitute a corresponding kind of screen; and any such
screen necessarily directs the attention to one field rather than another" (*Language* 50). By examining the different terministic screens that permeate our
interaction in human society, we can trace how each kind of screen "le[ads]
to a correspondingly different quality of observations" (49). Those different
observations, in turn, shape our relations with each other as symbolic agents.

The terministic screens of biomedical practitioners are shaped largely by
an idiom of disease, within which patient care is predicated on the scientific
model. Practitioners' expert knowledge enables them to re-present patients'
subjective illness experiences in seemingly objective medical terms as a diagnosis (Cicourel; Hunter), and their treatments are also generally limited to
that same idiom. Patients are not so restricted, however, and many will try
a variety of treatments, particularly those for whom mainstream medicine
has not provided much relief. Their terministic screens—the terms in which
they see and understand their bodies, their health, and their health care—
are determined more significantly by the experience of illness, including pain,
suffering, fear, limited ability, interpersonal strain, and financial loss. That is,
while the terministic screens of biomedical practitioners "direct the attention"

toward explanations of disease as essentially organic, rooted in biological pathology, patients' screens direct the attention toward how that disease plays out within individual bodies and lives. In the context of CAM, biomedical practitioners might, for example, dismiss an intervention such as chiropractic because its purported mechanism of action, the correction of spinal misalignment or "subluxation," does not fit with their own theoretical "screens," while patients may instead be concerned only about whether it will alleviate their pain or help them regain enough mobility to return to work.

Medical anthropologist Arthur Kleinman frames this disjunction between physician and patient perspectives as a problem of "conflicting explanatory models." Explanatory models, Kleinman explains, are mental schemes for organizing and understanding the various dimensions of illness, particularly as they pertain to clinical decision-making. For any given episode of illness, there are several explanatory models—the doctor's, the patient's, the patient's family's—each of which may sponsor different courses of action. Explanatory models work as "justifications for practical action more than statements of a theoretical or rigorous nature" (121), whereas terministic screens, I would argue, produce exactly the latter sort of theoretical or rigorous statement. As justifications for action, explanatory models are therefore more pliable than terministic screens because they are fundamentally pragmatic, oriented to action, and can more easily be understood by those who do not hold them. Terministic screens instead shape the very ways that we "see" a given situation: we cannot see what is blocked by our terminology from view.

These two ways of understanding physician and patient perspectives can help unpack some of the rhetorical complexity of practitioner-patient interaction because, although the two frameworks overlap significantly, they highlight different dimensions of the clinical exchange. Terministic screens can illuminate deeply held conceptual understandings of a given health problem (e.g., what it is, what it means), while explanatory models can reveal participants' somewhat more flexible beliefs about what to *do* about that problem. Phrased another way, while explanatory models determine what we think *about* in health care contexts (such as courses of action), terministic screens determine what we think *with*.

To return to the example of chiropractic's theoretical mechanism of action, physicians might not be able to identify with their patients' interest in seeing a chiropractor because their biomedical training screens from view the possibility that spinal subluxation contributes to illness. However, by eliciting their patients' explanatory models of their conditions, physicians might better come to appreciate the reasons for that interest and therefore better

negotiate courses of treatment. The reverse is true as well: patients not limited to a biomedical screen may not identify with their physicians' skepticism
about chiropractic but, if privy to medicine's explanatory models, they might
more easily accept that skepticism as rooted in valid reasoning, which could
also influence treatment decisions.

Although Kleinman does not himself ascribe a rhetorical function to explanatory models, he nevertheless shows that they can persuade—and fail to
persuade, as happens frequently in the care of chronic illness. For example,
the physician who does not explain the particulars of his or her own medical
explanatory model, who takes that model as already known and accepted by
the patient, will fail to persuade the chronically ill person in search of a cure
about the limits of medical treatment. Similarly, the physician who does not
take seriously the patient's explanatory model of his or her own illness risks
alienating the patient and "undermin[ing] the communicative foundations
of care" (122).[5] This is the thinking that underlies the "concordance" model
of care, the rhetoric of which holds that, unlike the compliance model where
patients are expected to follow "doctor's orders," patient preferences and beliefs must be taken into account in clinical decision-making.

Patient perspectives often receive short shrift in biomedicine, where
priority is generally accorded to physicians, who hold a wealth of cultural
capital. This capital is transformed into linguistic capital through the generic
structures of medicine itself, such as the regulated, and regulating, ways in
which doctor-patient encounters unfold. Kleinman illustrates how clinical
encounters can be particularly troubling for patients with chronic conditions
because their experience of illness, itself a form of expertise, is routinely overlooked by physicians who interrupt and redirect patients attempts' to convey
their explanatory models. Such interruptions and redirections, Kleinman
suggests, derive from the physician's effort to glean the information that his
biomedical explanatory model deems most salient, in effect (but unintentionally) crowding the patient out of her own care. In such cases, Kleinman
notes, the physician ultimately conveys to patients the message that "your
view doesn't really matter much; I am the one who will make the treatment
decisions; you do not need to be privy to the influences and judgments that
inform those decisions" (130). For patients with nonspecific symptoms (pain,
fatigue) or chronic illness, the discounting of their own embodied expertise
not only compromises the quality of their care—it may lead them to seek care
elsewhere.

The discursive shape of a practice such as chiropractic diverges radically
from the model of physician-centric interaction that Kleinman describes.
While biomedical patients are expected to adapt to the physician's explana-

tory model, there is in chiropractic a stronger impulse to bridge the gap between the perspectives of practitioner and patient. Kaptchuk and Eisenberg,
the Harvard Medical School-based CAM researchers, argue, for example, that:

> Chiropractic finds its voice exactly where biomedicine becomes inarticulate.
> Too often, biomedicine fails to affirm a patient's chronic pain. Patients think
> their experience is brushed aside by a physician who treats it as unjustified,
> unfounded, or annoying, attitudes that heighten a patient's anguish and in-
> tensify suffering. . . . Chiropractic's ultimate lesson may be to reinforce the
> principle that the patient-physician relationship is fundamentally about words
> and deeds of connection and compassion. ("Chiropractic" 2221–22)

Framing Kaptchuk and Eisenberg's observation in Kleinman's terms, chiropractic excels at something that biomedicine generally does not: affirming,
and even working within, the patients' own explanatory models.

The overall tenor of chiropractic is more relational than instrumental,
particularly after the initial consultation phase. In her research on communication at a chiropractic clinic, Oths found, for example, that once the treatment protocol had been identified, practitioner-patient exchanges became
increasingly more affective, with the chiropractor asking after patients' home
and work lives as he performed his spinal adjustments ("Communication" 93).
This discreet, "amiable chatting" about patients' lives is not, in Oths's view,
meant simply to pass the time while the practitioner administers his physical
treatment ("Unintended" 107). Rather, she suggests, affective talk in chiropractic operates, often unintentionally, as what Kleinman et al. call "a culturally
disguised form of psychotherapy" (qtd. in Oths, "Unintended" 88).

The ongoing clinical relationship, maintained primarily through affective
talk, is, in Oths's view, the key to patients' higher levels of satisfaction and
to chiropractic's perceived efficacy. Her explanation of the therapeutic functions of affective talk runs along several axes: that affective talk helps to address the psychosomatic dimensions of chronic conditions such as back pain
and headache; that it increases patients' feelings of control over their illnesses
and environments; that it provides vital social support by instilling a sense
of hope and encouragement; and that it makes patients feel integral to their
own care rather than passive recipients of it. What Oths does not spell out in
the course of her analyses, however, is that all of these dimensions of care are
also importantly persuasive.

Implicit in Oths's analysis is the suggestion that chiropractic care's affective, relational effects may enhance patients' compliance and continued treatment, although she stops short of suggesting that practitioners may capitalize
on their patients' explanatory models, if unwittingly. However, by discussing

patients' health within the context of their work lives (e.g., "Did you change shifts yet?" "Did you get your raise?") and home lives ("How were the holidays?" "Did you talk it over with your wife?"), chiropractors do (at least) two things at once: they affirm patients' lived experience of chronic illness within the context of their everyday lives, which serves a therapeutic function; and they affirm their own position as a practitioner that "cares" and "listens," serving their own professional interests by securing the continued patronage of patients attracted to those aspects of care.[6] While it may not be an explicit or conscious strategy, affective talk in the chiropractic clinic may, then, be as much a part of chiropractic's sales pitch as it is a part of its model of care.

One potential drawback of incorporating high levels of affective communication into chiropractic, as Oths points out, is that it could put patients on the defensive by imputing a psychosomatic dimension to their condition—as if to say, "there's nothing wrong, it's all in your head" ("Unintended" 108). However, this affective dimension of care seems to be enabled largely by the rhetorical work accomplished in the initial consultation phase. Chiropractic care typically involves an "intake" phase at the start of a clinical relationship, to assess the patient's orthopedic health through range-of-motion tests, visual assessment, questionnaires, x-rays, and scans, and to outline a treatment plan in consultation with the patient. Education about chiropractic theory is also central to this process. Major chiropractic concepts are demonstrated on patients' bodies and models (usually replica spines and joints), as well as through films, posters, and handouts, all of which promote a chiropractic understanding of health and illness. This rapid and intense orientation to care seems effectively to align the patient's explanatory model with that of the practitioner. Through this process, Oths concludes, "In essence, the chiropractor first manipulates a patient's belief structure before setting about to manipulate his or her physical structure. . . . A congruity between patient beliefs and behaviors gives a certain unity to the chiropractic experience, securing patient faith in and adherence to the system of therapy" ("Communication" 91).

There seems, then, to be a double shift in chiropractic, where the patient's beliefs about her condition and her expectations for treatment are given priority in their own right *and* are brought into closer alignment with practitioner's explanatory model, even though their underlying, theoretically oriented terministic screens may remain distinct. The distinction between explanatory models and terministic screens is important here because it makes it possible for a patient to believe in the practical effects of an intervention without necessarily subscribing to its more deeply seated philosophical foundations. For example, a patient can believe in the idea that manipulating the skeletal structure can restore mobility and improve health (an explanatory model) without believing in chiropractic's underlying concept of "Innate Intelligence" (a terministic screen), the God-like force professed to be released with the correction of subluxation (Keating 79). This double shift in chiropractic care, which harmonizes practitioner and patient explanatory models, seems to create fertile ground for a productive, ongoing therapeutic relationship by fostering between chiropractor and patient what rhetorician Chaim Perelman calls a "meeting of minds." Without such a meeting of minds, no persuasion is possible.[7]

When chiropractic is adapted to research contexts, these efforts at practitioner-patient alignment are absent: the comprehensive intake procedures standard in chiropractic care are not typically replicated in clinical trials and the therapeutic potential of practitioner-patient interaction is controlled for by means such as standardization and blinding. The trials may consequently inhibit the development of that crucial common ground between practitioner and patient, which Oths links directly (though not wholly) to chiropractic's efficacy. In the *JAMA* theme issue, Bove and Nilsson, for example, compared spinal manipulation with a placebo laser treatment for headache, emphasizing that the treatment arms were indistinguishable beyond the isolated spinal adjustment. As in the other RCTs in the *JAMA-Archives* theme issues on CAM (e.g., Cardini and Weixin; Shlay et al.), this study appears to have placed participants into assigned groups without providing further background or theoretical information on the interventions they would receive, and so the studies overlook the role that a meeting of minds, established in those crucial first chiropractic appointments, might play in the intervention's effects. Similarly, the authors rule out the evaluation of an affective or interactive dimension in chiropractic care by "controll[ing] for the treatment elements of personal attention and hands-on treatment" across both the intervention and control groups (1579). Identifying this design feature as one of the trial's strengths, Bove and Nilsson conclude that spinal manipulation is no more effective than placebo.

What Bove and Nilsson cite as one of their study's strongest features—that they have isolated spinal adjustment itself as the "active ingredient" in chiropractic care, with all other aspects of the trial arms identical—becomes a critical weakness within the domain of research on socially complex interventions. Such a view of chiropractic is troublingly reductive in its context as a "complex package of care" (Paterson and Dieppe) because spinal adjustment is usually complemented by a host of related activities, including individualized assessment, in-clinic and at-home exercises, lifestyle advice, interpersonal and affective talk, and touching.

Despite the difficulty of designing studies of practices such as chiropractic, importantly, research on CAM also seems to have the potential for an ameliorative effect on some of the more programmatic aspects of evidence-based medicine: trials of practices such as acupuncture and chiropractic have necessitated a number of methodological innovations that have led to more expansive discussions about how medical evidence is produced and for what purpose. One such example is the need to control for placebo effects, effects that occur in clinical trials when participants report or researchers observe improvement in the absence of an active intervention. The idea of the placebo effect as mere statistical noise, a product of overactive imaginations, is pervasive, often linked to what I have called the contaminating effects of practitioner-patient interaction. The placebo concept is being revisited in some quarters of medical research, particularly in recent studies of acupuncture. These studies highlight the importance of what were formerly considered, dismissively, the "nonspecific" aspects of care—aspects of care not linked directly to a known active ingredient. The investigation of placebo effects is beginning to offer new evidence on how practitioner-patient interaction can shape health outcomes, not only in CAM but in socially complex interventions more broadly, which may, in turn, begin to shift the boundaries of biomedicine itself.

Purifying Placebo Effects

The key requirement of a placebo control is that it must remain identical in all aspects to the study intervention with the exception of the active ingredient. In pharmaceutical trials, for instance, placebos are matched to the intervention drug in taste, color, size, texture, and dosing regimen, so that no one but the study's pharmacist need know to which trial arm any participant belongs. In an effectively controlled trial, with participants and researchers both unaware of treatment assignment, the results are unlikely to be contaminated by placebo effects, when the act of treatment itself affects the outcome. All participants would receive the same baseline "amount" of placebo, so that the effect of the active intervention could be measured differentially against the control group.

The problem, in socially complex interventions, is that separating out the "active ingredient" to create a lookalike dummy intervention is a conceptually impossible task. While a sugar pill can take on the appearance of a pharmacologically active pill without taking on its pharmacological activity, how does one feign the appearance of an "active ingredient" in a nursing intervention or a CAM practice when the precise nature of that active ingredient is unknown?

Further, supposing that practitioner-patient interaction could be isolated as the active ingredient, how would one devise a placebo of "interaction"—a sham intervention that takes on the appearance of interaction without consisting of actual interaction? Even if a placebo control could be devised for a trial of a given socially complex intervention, the placebo concept remains difficult to square with the individualized model of care characteristic of many such practices. Acupuncture, for instance, must be altered within research contexts: although acupuncturists engage in a patient-specific, evolving process of diagnosis and treatment, and although they consider their idiosyncratic skills and approaches essential to their efficacy as practitioners, these qualities of acupuncture care are difficult to standardize across multicenter trials.

Added to these problems of placebo-controlling studies of socially complex interventions are problems of blinding. The ideal clinical trial is double-blind, so that neither participants nor those administering the intervention know whether participants are receiving an active treatment or an inert control. The blinding of trial participants ("single-blinding") aims to head off anticipatory treatment effects, when participants' beliefs in or hopes for therapy register as real outcomes, while the blinding of trial staff ("double-blinding") aims both to prevent similar anticipatory effects in the observers and to protect against unintentional communication to participants of their group assignment. Manual therapies such as acupuncture and chiropractic pose difficulty for single-blinding because the practices involve interventions that are difficult to simulate with placebo procedures: in acupuncture, needles are inserted visibly into the skin, and in chiropractic, the spine is manipulated with a swift, physical, and often audible movement. Double-blinding is not possible because practitioners need to know whether or not to insert needles or move the spine. A further problem with blinding, as we saw in the previous chapter with the traditional Chinese medicine practitioner that I interviewed, Dr. Connolly, is that some practitioners consider their own intention to heal vital to their treatment's efficacy, and so double-blinding may not be desirable in such cases even if it were possible.

Various methods have been developed in acupuncture trials to try to get around the first problem, of finding plausible controls, but all introduce new problems. One approach is to use sham acupuncture, which employs either retractable needles that only appear to penetrate the skin or needles that are inserted into non-traditional points at shallow depths. However, nonpenetrating needles may not ensure concealment while non-traditional points may not be inert because the inserted needles might introduce new, untraceable effects of their own. Other options include active controls, which use the standard of care as a comparator (usually a pharmaceutical), and no-treatment controls, where participants in the control group receive no intervention at all, placebo or otherwise. However, these approaches eliminate the *relational* dimension of acupuncture, so they do not serve as proper placebo controls, narrowly construed, since the acupuncture-arm participants would receive more hands-on, interactive care.[8]

In terms of blinding, researchers can opt to conduct a single-blind study and have the outcomes assessed by an independent evaluator, to sidestep the possibility that those administering the intervention could anticipate treatment effects based on their knowledge of the participants' group assignment. However, even with an independent evaluation, the possibility remains that the acupuncturist could inadvertently communicate to the participant his or her group assignment and therefore jeopardize the results. Such a trial design is particularly risky for research on the boundaries of biomedicine because single-blinded studies sit lower on the hierarchies of evidence-based medicine than those that are double-blinded (see table 2 in chapter 3).

Evidence hierarchies are crucial in debates about whether or not a given practice is deemed safe and effective. Under the purview of evidence-based medicine, skeptics only need to call upon a higher standard of evidence to question or even dismiss an intervention under study. Recall, for instance, the response of Dr. Fournier, one of the research methodologists I cited in the previous chapter, who had been satisfied with the design of the Cardini and Weixin trial of moxibustion for the reversal of breech pregnancies until he discovered that the study's result had been positive. Upon reading the results section, he searched back through the article for possible flaws, calling upon an even higher standard in the design to explain how the study's outcome might be mistaken.

These sorts of methodological problems have frustrated researchers by limiting the validity of their results. With sham acupuncture, for instance, needling is isolated as the active ingredient and all other aspects of each arm remain equal (much like spinal adjustment in Bove and Nilsson's RCT of treatments for tension headache), but if the intervention's effects lie in one or more of those other aspects (described next), then the trial would not be able to pick up the difference. If indeed practitioner-patient interaction is a factor in acupuncture's efficacy, then trials that focus only on needling would be unable to trace those interactive effects because participants in each arm would experience the same quantity and quality of interaction. Such a design may easily lead to a false negative result (Paterson and Dieppe), wherein the lack of proof of an intervention's effect may be taken as proof of a lack of effect (Stener-Victorin et al.). Disputes about the validity of complementary and alternative medicine often invoke this line of reasoning, whereas few similar studies of nursing or unit-level interventions in hospitals would likewise be dismissed on these grounds.

Given the ease with which research on CAM can be dismissed on account of placebo effects, anxieties about avoiding such effects run high in the *JAMA-Archives* theme issues. In a brief news piece in *JAMA*, for example, Lynn Lamberg reports on the publication in the previous month's issue of *Archives of General Psychiatry* of several successful placebo-controlled studies of light therapy for winter seasonal affective disorder. Lamberg reports that one of the chief benefits of these studies is that they might help to rehabilitate the profession's view of light therapy, which had typically been regarded, in the view of one sleep researcher, as "not molecular enough, a bit too Californian-alternative, a bit too media overexposed, merely a placebo response by mildly neurotic middle-aged women who don't like nasty drugs" (qtd. in Lamberg 1558). What is interesting in this quotation is that the researcher's concern is not about whether or not light therapy has an effect—she takes the effect as given—but whether or not the explanation of that effect will persuade her science-minded biomedical colleagues. Will they see the effect of the intervention as real or imagined?

The idea of placebo effects as the product of overactive imaginations is pervasive in the *JAMA-Archives* theme issues, although not all commentators see this as a bad thing. In *Archives of Dermatology*, for example, dermatologist Francisco Tausk asks of alternative medicine: "Is it all in your mind?" Tausk surveys the current state of research on placebo or "nonspecific" effects of therapy—when "the specific effect of a drug or therapeutic modality is accompanied by nonspecific effects that may influence positively or negatively the outcome of the therapy" (1422). Tausk argues that nonspecific effects can and should be tested and implemented purposefully in practice. In the same journal, O'Sullivan, Lipper, and Lerner attempt to reframe the placebo concept by postulating a link between psychosocial factors and "neuro-immuno-cutaneous-endocrine" processes that affect the skin (1431). By explaining in thoroughly biomedical terms this mysterious phenomenon, when patients improve despite not having received any identifiable therapy, both sets of authors bridge the apparent conceptual divide between arguing for increased attention to (and even active solicitation of) placebo effects, on the one hand, and urging more rigorous, placebo-controlled studies of CAM on the other.

In the years immediately following the *JAMA-Archives* theme issues, researchers began in earnest to query the wisdom of the placebo control in research, suggesting that the quest to determine an intervention's "fastidious efficacy," its proof of efficacy under rigidly controlled conditions (Kaptchuk,

"Placebo Effect"), comes at the cost of its clinical significance. Further, these commentators argued that the notion of the placebo teaches patients (and their physicians) to be suspicious of their bodies and of their overall sense of wellness, thereby potentially undermining the health care they seek (see, e.g., Kaptchuk; Paterson and Dieppe). Patients who might otherwise relish feeling better may instead get tangled up in worries about whether they really are better, or just think they are better. Canadian columnist Stephen Strauss documents exactly this process when he writes of cortisone injections he had recently received: "But as I was starting to feel better I had a doubt: Was the relief due to real medicine or was I feeling merely the placebo effect? And what difference would that make? And what if painlessness were 20-per-cent placebo effect, 80-per-cent cortisone's healing power?"

The theoretical questions precipitated by the design problems of trials of acupuncture and other CAM interventions have prompted innovative new research on treatment effects more generally, fostering a greater appreciation of their variety. Rather than sending any and all sorts of "nonspecific effects" into the placebo wastebasket, this research and similar work in fields such as nursing (see Lindsay) has allowed researchers to consider the therapeutic potential of these effects and to develop multileveled trial designs that can get at some of their clinical nuances, rather than to try to control for them. This research is opening up promising new understandings of how patients respond to care, both as physical bodies and as persons. I want to suggest here that this is one way in which biomedical boundary work can have ameliorative effects on mainstream medicine, because the research conducted at the edges of biomedicine can feed back into the mainstream new perspectives on health and healing, on medical research and practice, and even on the culture of medicine itself.

The dichotomization of treatment effects as either *genuine* or *placebo* serves as a terministic screen that appears to greatly restrict other ways that researchers might understand the connections between health interventions and the conditions under which they operate. Although this division of effects in biomedical understandings of efficacy is widespread, much recent scholarship has indicated that it is "not meaningful to split complex interventions" this way (Paterson and Dieppe 1202; see also Kaptchuk, "Placebo Effect"). As a means to rehabilitate the placebo concept, Paterson and Dieppe frame this conventional division between real and imagined effects as instead a division between *characteristic* and *incidental* elements. In Paterson and Dieppe's framework, characteristic, or specific, effects include treatment factors that are both rooted in theory and causally linked with health outcomes, whereas incidental, or nonspecific, effects include "the many other factors that have also been shown to affect outcome, such as the credibility of the intervention, patient expectations, the manner and consultation style of the practitioner, and the therapeutic setting" (1202). For these researchers, the placebo concept is inadequate for explaining the many dimensions of how the act of care can itself affect patient outcomes, even in the absence of a clearly identified active intervention.

These and similar discussions have produced significant new models of biomedical research. For example, even the most prestigious medical journals such as the *Annals of Internal Medicine*, the *British Medical Journal*, *JAMA*, the *Lancet*, and the *New England Journal of Medicine* have featured essays extrapolating the problem of identifying placebo controls in CAM research to socially complex interventions more broadly construed.[9] Many of these models accord with what Nahin and Straus call the "whole system" approach (162), an approach that reinstalls interventions into their contexts of care, putting the whole package to the test rather than simply isolating the so-called active ingredient. Whole-systems approaches appear to shift the research enterprise dramatically by introducing within it principles of patient-centered care. Rather than testing acupuncture as though it were a pharmaceutical, for example, a whole-package approach would test needling alongside other traditional components of Chinese medicine, such as herbal therapies, cupping, dietary changes, exercise, moxibustion, massage, and sustained verbal and nonverbal interaction between practitioners and patients.

The new research models prompted by research on complementary and alternative medicine are grounded, conceptually, in a more textured view of the purpose and effects of medical research. In the UK Medical Research Council's guidelines on designing RCTs of socially complex interventions, for example, the council argues that trial design ought to limit the power of a single study to investigating only *whether* a complex practice is effective or *why* it is so, but not both. In asking whether a practice works, so-called fastidious design may actually hinder its application to practice because it would abstract pieces of the intervention from the whole. Breaking the intervention into parts could splinter or halt its effects. In the Bove and Nilsson study in the *JAMA* theme issue, for instance, spinal manipulation is isolated from all of the other factors characteristic of chiropractic, including affective care, even though, as Oths argues, affective care is likely one of the keys to chiropractic's perceived efficacy. A clinical study that does not factor interpersonal and interactive elements into its design may well fail to capture how that intervention works in practice.

In socially complex interventions, both in biomedicine and in CAM, the active treatment agent is unspecified, which complicates randomization in research settings. One solution would be to randomize at the level of the practitioner or clinic, rather than that of individual participants. The aim of such a design, according to van Weel and Knottnerus, would be to study the intervention's "gross clinical effect" rather than its constituent parts:

> This [new research] context brings back the generic, non-specific effects of the doctor-patient relationship that represent important interventions for the outcome of care. To designate those effects as a placebo effect . . . can remove such basic components from the evaluation by simply blinding or controlling for it. However, it is more appropriate to assess these effects in terms of the specific effects of interventions, and that is where a multilevel design can be helpful. (van Weel and Knottnerus 917–18)

Such a design reframes what I have called in this chapter "rhetorical interaction," all of the ways in which people act on and with one another as symbolic agents, as a key constituent of socially complex interventions rather than as a potential contaminant. This more expansive view of the practitioner-patient relationship has the potential to enhance the role of interaction effects in assessments of what counts as effective health care.

A 2008 study from the *British Medical Journal* offered an early signal that these new research models, which emerged partly out of the push for evidence on CAM in the early 1990s, had begun to bear fruit in the decade following the *JAMA-Archives* theme issues. In that study, Kaptchuk et al. investigated whether or not placebo effects could be divided, experimentally, into responses to three distinct elements of care: assessment and observation; a "therapeutic ritual (placebo treatment)"; and "a supportive practitioner-patient relationship" (999). The multilevel study's design sought to differentiate among these possible effects by increasing and combining them over time. The trial arms consisted of a wait list, a placebo treatment option (a nonpiercing sham acupuncture device) with limited practitioner-patient interaction (initial consult of no more than five minutes), and the same placebo treatment augmented with increased practitioner-patient interaction (initial consult of forty-five minutes, with the practitioner demonstrating "warmth," active listening, and concern for the patient's illness experience). The study's finding that nonspecific effects could indeed be divided into components and then combined in "graded dose escalation" corroborates the longtime claims of patient-centered care advocates that clinical interaction can itself have therapeutic value.

The study's conclusion that the practitioner-patient relationship is the "most robust" (999) of these components of the placebo effect is something of a triumph for commentators such as Feinstein and Horwitz, who worry that the significance of the clinical relationship may be lost in the sweep of evidence-based methods. For, if research verifies the importance of interaction on patient outcomes, then it stands to reason that the clinical relationship would be protected, and even bolstered, under the aegis of evidence-based medicine.[10] However, one could also argue that the *kind* of clinical relationship at the heart of patient-centered care is transformed beyond recognition just by virtue of its being installed within an experimental framework. Pat Bracken, for example, a psychiatrist with a PhD in philosophy, criticized the Kaptchuk trial for subjecting nonspecific treatment effects, including those of practitioner-patient interaction, to "the same positivist tools" used to study specific effects. In a follow-up letter, Kaptchuk accounted for such criticism by countering that, in an evidence-based culture, we can and must "be specific about non-specifics," regardless of how theoretically top-heavy such studies can be (Authors' Response). There is a certain incongruity in Kaptchuk's pragmatism here, as he advocates subjecting elements of care often considered beyond (and even antithetical to) the reaches of evidence-based methods to those very same methods. However, the risk that he and his coinvestigators take is calculated: the only sure means through which nonspecific effects in health care can assume significance in an evidence-based hierarchy is to validate them *within* that hierarchy.

In the context of biomedical boundary work, research on placebo and interactive effects, such as Kaptchuk et al.'s and later studies (see those cited in note 9 above but also Bishop et al.; Kaptchuk et al., "Maybe"), has several important but conflicting implications. On the one hand, the research widens the scope of clinical behaviors that may be deemed "effective," making space for relational or interactive effects alongside more straightforwardly tested interventions such as pharmaceuticals. This expanded scope for investigating clinical efficacy could have a limiting effect on arguments that seek to invalidate practices such as acupuncture and chiropractic on the ground that their efficacy derives from "mere" placebo effects. Additionally, research on placebo effects may improve patients' standing as medical and rhetorical subjects because it may make it harder to summarily dismiss nonspecific effects as imaginary, as the products of confused or gullible minds. Patients whose own bodily perceptions can more reliably be trusted make more persuasive patients. For example, if researchers argue that placebo effects are a "genuine psychobiological phenomenon" (Finniss et al.) and that they "should be maximized by harnessing patients' expectations . . . to improve treatment outcomes" (Enck et al. 191), suddenly the patient who responds to a treatment whose active ingredient is unknown seems a little less suspect, and perhaps even a little more reliable as a partner in care.

On the other hand, although studies such as Kaptchuk et al.'s help to affirm the importance of practitioner-patient interaction for clinical outcomes, they also appear to strengthen, and even expand, biomedical boundaries by affirming biomedicine's epistemic and professional jurisdiction over an (expanding) array of health-related matters. Kaptchuk et al.'s pragmatism about being "specific about nonspecifics" is necessary for their study to have credibility within the mainstream medical community. However, this pragmatism may come at high cost for both socially complex interventions and patient-centered care, both of which are vital to the evidence base for CAM: once placebo effects have been broken down into constituent parts, the argument for evaluating such interventions as whole "packages of care" may be harder to make, since each layer of the intervention might conceivably be peeled back and tested separately. The experimental isolation of specific dimensions of clinical care, and the subsequent validation of some and invalidation of others, could lead to the very same piecemeal or algorithmic approach to clinical practice for which evidence-based medicine has been heavily criticized. Experimental confirmation of the effects of "warmth" or "active listening," for example, could conceivably lead to clinical practice guidelines and checklists mandating the performance of these "proven" behaviors in patient consultations.

These potential concerns aside, the experimental validation of interaction effects as more than simply imaginary hooks into a larger movement in health research toward situating patient-centered modes of practice and evaluation within an evidence-based framework, the same movement within which biomedical research on CAM first gained its impetus. Patient-centered care's relentless focus on placing the patient, and not just his or her disease, at the center of the medical encounter can shift our attention from biomedical knowledge to the conditions of its production. Studies of CAM can be instructive for this shift because their methodological complexity makes the normally tacit procedures of medical research "strange," and therefore more readily open to inspection since there is no established method of proceeding. Tracking the decisions that researchers in the *JAMA-Archives* theme issues on CAM make as they design trials of practices such as chiropractic and acupuncture can tell us a lot about how the medical profession imagines the role and place of patients in both research and practice. By examining such studies, we can watch these boundary-negotiating processes unfold.

While Kaptchuk et al.'s point of entry in the new push for research on placebo and interactive effects is at the front end, through the conceptual work in the design phase to isolate distinct components of nonspecific effects, others have focused on the back end, where innovations lie not so much in design but in evaluation, such as developing more appropriate assessment tools or outcome measures (e.g., Ritenbaugh). According to Paul Dieppe, a physician-researcher who has become an authority on trial design for complex interventions, the key to assessing nonspecific effects in an evidence-based framework is to consider carefully what sorts of questions the research means to ask and determine how best to design the study to answer those questions. Dieppe proposes a suite of prospective trial designs that may open up new lines of inquiry into the range of effects currently defined as nonspecific, contextual, or placebo effects. Projects such as Dieppe's represent a major shift in thinking about the place of patients within health research because they aim to tweak the RCT format into a model more amenable to aspects of care not easily captured in conventional studies.

Even in the face of methodological innovation, however, patient-centered approaches to research fit only awkwardly within the realm of medical practice, whether that practice is evidence-based or not. Moreover, when examined more closely, evidence-based medicine and patient-centered care are compatible in perhaps surprising ways—ways not only that enable the development of a hybrid model, evidence-based patient choice (Edwards and Elwyn), but also that constrain it. In biomedical boundary work, this new model may serve as a template for doctor-patient consultations about CAM, particularly given that a central tension in the *JAMA-Archives* theme issues is whether and how physicians should (or even can) advise patients about complementary and alternative medicine. As a template for interaction, the next section argues, the model of evidence-based patient choice helps us to track some of the potential implications of biomedical research on CAM for conventional medical practice and the ability of evidence on practitioner-patient interaction to determine the boundaries of biomedicine.

Patient Choice across Medical Models

To return to Epstein et al.'s definition of patient-centered care cited in this chapter's introduction, this construct is predicated on the idea that providing health care "concordant with the patient's values, needs and preferences" will ultimately improve the overall health of persons. A large body of research indicates that patient-centered methods do result in material gains for many patients, particularly in studies that foreground practitioner-patient communication (Ong et al.; Stewart; Stewart and Brown). However, I argue in this section that the applicability of patient-centered care is less assured under the rhetorical conditions governing clinical practice than its proponents suggest. That is, there seems to be some slippage between patient-centered care as a theoretical model and the enactment of that model in practice, a slippage that I suggest here is particularly true of complementary and alternative medicine because "choice," in many CAM practices, may be more illusory than real.

Emphasis in patient-centered care on the patient as an equal partner and decision maker does not mesh well with biomedicine's institutional-professional discursive practices, which frame patients as ultimately scenic, in Kenneth Burke's terms—as containers of disease and sites of treatment rather than as autonomous agents (*Grammar*; see also Martha Solomon). These discursive processes operate systemically in biomedicine: through genre, as rhetoricians Schryer and Spoel have shown with the formation of medical-professional identities; through clinical conversation between medical experts and nonexperts, as linguist Elisabeth Gülich has shown; and through lexicogrammatical processes of enculturation, as physician Perri Klass has shown of medical training. On all of these discursive levels, patients are situated firmly as the objects and subjects of medicine, not as agents within it.

Consider, for instance, Sarah Freymann Fontenot's account in *Physician Executive* of the US-based Patient-Centered Outcomes Research Institute (PCORI), which she explains was established in 2010 under the Affordable Care Act to improve "how physicians treat chronic disease and how patients participate in their own medical decision-making" (98). For PCORI, according to Fontenot, "The organizing theme is that not all treatments are effective, and *not all patients are appropriate for all treatments*" (98; emphasis added). For a patient-centered model of effectiveness research, PCORI's mandate in the italicized portion of this description is fully treatment-centered, organized not around patient needs but around administration of care. The phrasing of this description is more than superficial: it reflects deeply held, structural assumptions about the place of patients in medical care, even in contexts where the patient is ostensibly valued as a decision maker. As Judy Segal observes, a model of care that equalizes doctors and patients in decision-making "charges patients both to seek advice and to decide whether to take it, while the resources to make the decision may be locked inside the advice itself" (*Health* 144). Such a model, she explains, "presumes that physicians who otherwise continue to work in an old paradigm are able to equip patients as decision makers in a new one" (145). Making medicine more patient-centered is, therefore, a matter of more than simply giving doctors lessons in effective communication. More importantly, it would necessitate substantial conceptual shifts in medical research, funding, training, policy, implementation, and reimbursement.

Patient-centered care is difficult to square with medical practice from the perspective of patients as well: not all patients want to be in charge of their own health care, and some want to have only limited input in decision-making. For example, nearly a third of patients in one study preferred directive care over patient-centered, particularly older patients and those with life-threatening conditions (Swenson et al.). Part of the problem with the patient-as-decision-maker model of practice is that it applies an essentially economic metaphor to medicine, basing its emphasis on rational choice on a free market model in which "the typical autonomous agent seems like a sovereign customer with a coherent shopping list and a fat wallet in a well-stocked market" (qtd. in Elwyn and Edwards 3; see also Mol). But when patients seek health care, whether it is mainstream or alternative, they are not dispassionately shopping for groceries—they are seeking expertise, whether for advice, authorization, or treatment. And they seek that expertise within a power imbalance, under which the notion of choice might represent, to some, a kind of abandonment. Autonomy might, under this valence, erode trust and compromise individuals' feelings of control and confidence over their states of health.

Counterintuitively, the patient-as-decision-maker model may be problematic even for individuals who want to actively participate in their health care. Patients with chronic, functional conditions, who make up the majority of CAM users, may especially value a model of practice that places them squarely in charge of their own care but, even then, the actual degree of autonomy afforded may be less than advertised. In both biomedicine and CAM, the extent to which patient-centered care really is about the patient is open to question and may instead be largely about better disposing the patient, through a dynamic interplay, to follow medical advice. As Segal argues ("'Compliance,'" *Health*), concordance is touted as a model of collaborative decision-making but is essentially a dressed-up version of compliance, the paternalistic model of following "doctor's orders." As she points out, the goal even in concordance models remains to persuade patients to adhere to prescribed courses of treatment. Indeed, the very ability to offer choices at all invokes a kind of rhetorical authority unavailable to patients and bespeaks a residual doctor-knows-best mentality at work in even the most egalitarian of consultations.

As key terms, "patient-centeredness," "choice," and "autonomy" figure prominently in discussions of complementary and alternative medicine, but the possibility that a patient could choose wrongly is equally pervasive. Writing in the *JAMA* theme issue, for example, Sugarman and Burk urge doctors to practice shared decision-making with their patients who choose CAM, but they maintain that it is ultimately incumbent upon doctors to persuade their patients to make the right choices—to lead them, that is, toward "accepted" and "legitimate" health-related goals (1624; 1625). The same mentality of needing to direct patients in their decision-making appears to be true for some CAM practitioners as well. For example, Oths argues that chiropractors steer patients away from "unacceptable behaviors" through positive reinforcement and covert psychotherapy ("Unintended" 108). I would argue, further, that the very idea that a patient's behavior would require the practitioner's "acceptance" runs counter to the rhetorics of self-determination and nonjudgmental care that characterize CAM practices such as chiropractic.

Much of what looks like choice in chiropractic may not, in the end, stem from mutual decision-making between practitioner and patient, but from the chiropractor employing explanatory frameworks persuasively. Within the restricted purview of a given explanatory framework, a patient's sense of herself as an equal participant might be to a great extent illusory, as certain choices come to seem natural and inevitable—not as *preferred* options but as the *only* ones. I argued earlier in this chapter that the intake phase of chiropractic, when practitioners offer detailed chiropractic education and patient assessment, creates fertile ground for persuasion because it helps to establish common ground between practitioners and patients. This is the sense in which professionalized CAM practices such as chiropractic and acupuncture may not be as patient-centered as their accompanying discourses imply, because what looks like patient choice and autonomy is often more paternalistic than it first appears.[11] As Segal explains, "This is not to say that the *appearance* of consultation-between-equals would not be a good persuasive strategy. But, in some cases, a strategy is all it would be" (" 'Compliance' " 88).

Power is not native to patients in any medical setting, at least initially: patients approach the medical encounter from a vulnerable position as individuals in need of help and expertise. Enthusiastic appraisals of patient autonomy often fail to notice the irony that autonomy must be granted by an authorizing source. In health care contexts, this means that even if patients are viewed as autonomous decision makers, it is only because a higher authority has authorized such a view. In the CAM-themed issue of *Archives of Dermatology*, Robert Thomsen takes exactly this approach in instructing physicians to "give your patient permission to pursue other forms of health care" (1446). Most patients will seek CAM anyway, he argues, so granting permission allows physicians to remain within the circle of care. Of course, Thomsen's observation also illustrates that practitioners do not hold all of the power, either: physicians can urge courses of treatment, order laboratory tests, and write prescriptions, but, except in exceptional situations, patients can opt out at any stage of the process. Granting patients "permission" to use CAM, then, may in some cases be no more than a strategy to regain authority over patient care by granting patients a limited form of autonomy.

To facilitate patient autonomy in the context of medical research, numerous scholars and practitioners have recently advocated bringing evidence-based medicine and patient-centered care into a more formally integrated model of care, known as evidence-based patient choice (EBPC). This model's proponents maintain that EBPC combines the best of the two approaches, and to some extent this is true. Elwyn and Edwards note, for instance, that the kind of choice evinced in the patient-centered care literature can be "perversely impossible to manage" (9), and so, by couching the available options within the evidence base, practitioners can offer fewer yet potentially more effective interventions for patients to choose from. However, this new model is not so much a step forward in thinking about the connections between medical research and practice, particularly regarding CAM and other socially complex interventions, as it is a sign that the thinking has stalled. To the extent that health research agendas have expanded beyond a narrowly biomedical purview, the problems that remain are amplified within the more expansive, hybrid theoretical context of EBPC.

As in patient-centered care, for example, *choice* in this model is frequently anything but a matter of choice. Ford, Schofield, and Hope maintain that EBPC entails "providing patients with evidence-based information in a way that facilitates their ability to make choices or decisions about their health care" (589), but as Segal has shown, decisions within such a framework are not necessarily made freely. The manner in which choices are presented— their "framing effect" (Ashcroft, Hope, and Parker 61)—can, for example, render patients more likely to choose some options over others, simply based on how they are presented. These framing effects are particularly powerful when taken in the context of the rhetorical dynamics of practitioner-patient consultations, where even the most egalitarian of practitioners holds the balance of power by virtue of her expert authority—her ability to diagnose and treat illness.

Choice is limited further upstream in EBPC as well, at the level of evidence production, which again poses significant challenges for biomedical research on CAM, such as the research reported in the *JAMA-Archives* theme issues. One of the reasons that Ashcroft, Hope, and Parker give for why practitioners might legitimately refuse patients their choice of intervention is that "what the patient wants is futile—the treatment is ineffective" (57). But this reasoning simplifies the complex process of determining efficacy, a contingent exercise that the previous chapter illustrated is, in part, explicitly rhetorical. Randomized controlled trials of CAM are particularly contingent because the evidence they produce is necessarily provisional by virtue of their intractable design challenges. And yet, when that evidence is translated into clinical practice guidelines and insurance reimbursement schemes, it is reified in the process, becoming the firm ground upon which a slate of patient choices is formulated. A potential consequence of this reification of evidence is that, while a given patient may find relief in the nonspecific effects of chiropractic care, chiropractic may not be included among the options suggested by her family physician, on the basis that there is not enough evidence to support its use. The choice would in this sense have been made even prior to the clinical encounter, and not by the patient.

Further upstream still, the idea that research would directly inform practice is simply not borne out in studies of implementation, as discussed in chapter 3: there is often a poor association between the evidence base and clinical behavior, not only for research on CAM but even for research on many of the most widely used biomedical interventions. The assumption that research findings produced by clinical trials would translate directly into practice naively underestimates the complex negotiations that clinicians must undergo to assess competing bodies of data, including clinical experience, professional habits and competition, commercial interests, research evidence, clinical practice guidelines, and insurance schemes. For time-pressed doctors who do not always have the necessary background in reading the medical literature, research evidence may not always be accorded the status in practice that researchers and proponents of evidence-based medicine take for granted.

The "*JAMA* Patient Page" offered at the back of the 1998 theme issue, "Alternative Choices: What it Means to Use Nonconventional Medical Therapy" (see fig. 2), offers a glimpse into how a model of evidence-based patient choice could play out in advising patients about CAM. Meant to be photocopied and distributed to patients, the handout offers an extended definition of "alternative medicine" and brief descriptions of six of the more common CAM therapies (acupuncture, aromatherapy, chiropractic, folk medicine, herbal medicine, and homeopathy). In a sidebar, the handout features a list of "Issues to Consider about Alternative Therapies" (Hwang), which includes "Safety and effectiveness," "The Practitioner's Expertise," "Quality of Service Delivery," "Costs," and "Consult your Physician." Below this list are contact information for the National Institutes of Health's Office of Alternative Medicine and links to *JAMA*'s Patient Page website.[12]

Although the list of "Issues to Consider" appears to facilitate patient decision-making, it situates that process within a paternalistic relationship: the physician sets up the range of options from which the patient will choose. Further, patients are instructed to "[d]etermine if the delivery of service adheres

Alternative choices
What it means to use nonconventional medical therapy

ALTERNATIVE MEDICINE

If you've ever taken high-dose vitamins, used an herbal remedy, or sought treatment from a chiropractor, you're among the millions all over the world who use alternative medicine to ward off illness or treat a variety of ailments.

Known by a variety of terms – *complementary, holistic, unorthodox, integrative* – alternative medicine refers to most treatment practices that are not considered conventional medicine (widely practiced or accepted by the mainstream medical community). Although the majority of medicine practiced in the United States is conventional, worldwide, approximately 70% to 90% of health care is delivered by what would be considered an alternative tradition or practice.

Incorporating hundreds of different philosophies and procedures, alternative therapies are usually ideologically based. Most of these therapies often are not backed by scientific research that measures safety or effectiveness. Some alternative therapies have dangerous side effects. Another concern is that people who use alternative therapies in the place of conventional medical therapy may delay or lose the opportunity to benefit from scientifically based treatment.

The use of alternative medicine in the United States is growing in popularity.

According to a new study in the November 11, 1998, *JAMA* theme issue on alternative medicine, 4 out of 10 Americans use some form of alternative medicine. Americans visited alternative therapy practitioners 629 million times in 1997, a 47% increase over the 427 million visits made in 1990. They spent approximately $27 billion out-of-pocket (not covered by insurance) on alternative therapies in 1997, which is about the same as estimated 1997 out-of-pocket spending for all U.S. physician services.

Additional Sources: National Institutes of Health's Office of Alternative Medicine, AMA's Reader's Guide to Alternative Health Methods, American Cancer Society

ISSUES TO CONSIDER ABOUT ALTERNATIVE THERAPIES:

- **Safety and effectiveness** – The product or practice should not cause any harm and should provide benefit when used as intended. Specific information about the safety and effectiveness of any alternative or complementary therapy should be readily available.
- **The practitioner's expertise** – Closely examine the training, qualifications, and competence of any potential health care practitioner. Alternative medicine is not as well regulated as conventional medicine.
- **Quality of service delivery** – Determine if the delivery of service adheres to standards for medical safety and care; contact state or local regulatory agencies or health care consumer organizations; visit the practitioner's office, clinic, or hospital; and talk to people who have used the service.
- **Costs** – Many alternative therapies are not covered by health insurance, so compare the costs with those of other practitioners or through professional medical associations.
- **Consult your physician** – Discuss any type of medical therapy with your doctor. Your doctor needs to know about any conventional and alternative therapies you have used or are currently using to treat you more effectively and to prevent medication interactions.

SOME TYPES OF ALTERNATIVE MEDICINE:

- **Acupuncture** – Insertion of needles into specific points in the body for therapeutic purposes; also may involve use of heat, pressure, or electromagnetic energy to stimulate anatomic acupuncture points in the body
- **Aromatherapy** – Use of essential oils extracted from flowers, leaves, stalks, fruits, and roots for therapeutic purposes
- **Chiropractic** – Based on the idea that spinal misalignments are the principal cause of disease; uses manual procedures and interventions to manipulate the spine
- **Folk medicine** – Medical treatment based on the beliefs, traditions, or customs of a particular society or ethnic/cultural group

- **Herbal medicine** – Use of various parts of plants to treat symptoms and promote health; herbs have a long history in medicine, but many herbs that have been proven to be effective years ago have been replaced by more effective synthetic compounds; the U.S. Food and Drug Administration (FDA) does not currently regulate herbal products, and herbal products can only be marketed as dietary supplements because manufacturers and distributors cannot make any specific health claims without FDA approval
- **Homeopathy** – Remedies made from plant, animal, or mineral substances that are highly diluted with the intent to stimulate the body only enough to trigger a healing response

FOR MORE INFORMATION:

- National Institutes of Health
  Office of Alternative Medicine (OAM)
  OAM Clearinghouse
  (does not provide referrals or medical advice)
  P.O. Box 8218
  Silver Spring, MD 20910
  888/644-6226
  (8:30 a.m. to 5 p.m. ET weekdays)
  888/644-6226 (TTY) or altmed.od.nih.gov

INFORM YOURSELF:

To find this and previous *JAMA* Patient Pages, check out the AMA's Web site at www.ama-assn.org/consumer.htm.

COPY FOR YOUR PATIENTS!

Mi Young Hwang, Writer   Richard M. Glass, MD, Editor   Jeff Molter, Director of Science News

The JAMA Patient Page is a public service of JAMA and the AMA. The information and recommendations appearing on this page are appropriate in most instances; but they are not a substitute for medical diagnosis. For specific information concerning your personal medical condition, JAMA and AMA suggest that you consult your physician. This page may be reproduced noncommercially by physicians and other health care professionals to share with patients. Any other reproduction is subject to AMA approval. Bulk reprints available by calling 212/354-0050.

FIGURE 2. Patient handout from *Journal of the American Medical Association*: Mi Young Hwang, "Alternative Choices: What it Means to Use Nonconventional Medical Therapy [*JAMA* Patient Page]," *Journal of the American Medical Association* 280.18 (1998): 1640.

to standards for medical safety and care" for a particular CAM practice or practitioner, but, as nonmedical personnel, patients may not properly be equipped to evaluate such standards. Similarly, the handout informs patients that "Specific information about the safety and effectiveness of any alternative or complementary therapy should be readily available," but, as I have shown in previous chapters, that information is difficult even for medical practitioners to obtain and interpret, let alone for patients.

Ultimately, the first four items on the handout's list of "Issues to Consider" point to the fifth: "Discuss any type of medical therapy with your doctor. Your doctor needs to know about any conventional and alternative therapies you have used or are currently using to treat you more effectively and to prevent medication interactions" (Hwang). The framing effects of this document as a whole position the physician as the arbiter of the decision-making process, confirming Segal's findings that, in discourses about "concordance," a process that appears to belong primarily to the patient depends instead upon the physician's expert judgment.

The "*JAMA* Patient Page" gives some indication of how physicians might envision the shape of future patient consultations about CAM, in which such potentially boundary-crossing encounters would unfold with the physician firmly in charge. From the perspective of patients, however, many of whom seek CAM to regain a greater sense of agency in their health care, the shift toward a doctor-approved iteration of CAM might not be desirable. Moreover, as I have argued in this section, even CAM practices such as acupuncture and chiropractic may sometimes be too restrictive for patients seeking a sense of control over their health because their practitioners' emphases on patient choice and autonomy may be illusory, a means of seeking agreement with health-care choices that were effectively made even before they were offered. As I argue in the next section, we might, then, usefully think of consumption of dietary supplements as an extreme case of patient choice, one in which users partially opt out of professionalized health care, whether alternative or not. The rhetorical appeal of dietary supplements, I argue, rests largely on their promise of greater agency for patients, now as consumers. Consequently, discourses surrounding dietary supplements can further illuminate the ways in which patients are positioned as medical-rhetorical subjects in biomedical research on complementary and alternative medicine.

Dietary Supplements and Patient Agency

As a regulatory category, *dietary supplements* encompass health-related products taken orally that are not under the purview of the US Food and Drug

Administration (FDA). These products include high-dose vitamins, botanical remedies (including herbs), amino acids, and "substances such as enzymes, organ tissues, glandulars and metabolites" (Nisly et al.). Supplements range from highly concentrated forms of everyday foods such as garlic and ginger to pharmacologically active and potentially dangerous substances such as ephedra and valerian root. Various CAM practitioners prescribe dietary supplements, as do some physicians (although certainly fewer), but supplements are far more readily accessed without prescription through natural health food stores and, increasingly, pharmacies, grocery stores, and online retailers. Supplements are among the most highly accessed CAM modalities, more than any practitioner-administered modality including chiropractic and traditional Chinese medicine. In 2002, the Centers for Disease Control found that, after prayer, dietary supplements were the most-used CAM therapy by percentage of US adults in a twelve-month period, at 19 percent, while chiropractic, the highest-ranked professionalized practice, ranked seventh at 7.5 percent (Barnes et al.). A more recent US Department of Health and Human Services survey from 2007 found that 44 percent of all out-of-pocket expenses for CAM went toward dietary supplements, with spending just under one-third of that for all pharmaceutical drugs by Americans during the same period (Nahin et al.).

In the *JAMA* theme issue, a team led by David Eisenberg reported the results of a 1997 survey of CAM use and expenditure in the United States (Eisenberg et al., "Trends"), a follow-up to Eisenberg's landmark 1990 national survey (Eisenberg et al., "Unconventional"). The newer survey showed that, although Americans' use of supplements had already been widespread by the time of the earlier survey, that number had risen rapidly over seven years. Use of herbal remedies had risen 380 percent during that period and that of high-dose vitamins, 130 percent. Despite such high levels of use, the newer Eisenberg study also found that fewer than 40 percent of all CAM users reported that use to their doctors ("Trends" 1575). In the decade since the second Eisenberg study, levels of supplement use have risen even further, resulting not only in staggering sales (over $21 billion in 2006) but also in widespread concern about potential overuse and "polyherbacy," when individuals take concurrently multiple, possibly interacting, supplements or supplements and pharmaceuticals (Nisly et al.).[13] Because so few patients disclose their use of supplements to their physicians, interactions are a very real threat to patient safety and care.

One reason why such great numbers of patients choose to take dietary supplements is to gain a greater sense of control over their health within a medical system that is sometimes rhetorically disabling. As I have argued above, patients often struggle as interlocutors within the generic conventions of clinical practice. Supplements, by contrast, appear to place individuals in control of their own health care because, as consumers, they require neither a prescription nor permission to purchase and use products that they believe will enhance their health. Such a view is borne out by empirical research: anthropologists Nichter and Thompson's 2006 ethnographic study of supplement users indicated that the key factor in their participants deciding to take supplements either alongside or instead of conventional treatments was precisely because they felt that, in taking supplements, they gained greater agency over their own health care.

Questions surrounding patient agency run through the *JAMA-Archives* theme issues. In *JAMA*, for instance, Mike Mitka jokes that "Perhaps opponents and skeptics of the safety and efficacy of medicinal herbs should take echinacea to improve their immune systems so they can ward off the growing deluge of requests from consumers for these alternative medicines" (1554). Mitka's comment is cheeky, but it also speaks to an underlying concern within the medical profession about shifts in the doctor-patient dynamic as patients place increasing demands on physicians, who formerly held a position of privilege by virtue of their specialized knowledge and the generic constraints of doctor-patient interaction.

Mitka cites Loren Israelsen, executive director of the Utah Natural Products Alliance, who argues that the issue of dietary supplements has moved beyond questions of *whether* patients should be using them to questions of *when* and *how*: "Consumers are voting with their feet, and that makes some in the medical profession unhappy. . . . These medical professionals say, 'They should be coming to me instead of going to their pharmacists or health food store.' But patients say they would visit their physicians if the physicians knew something about these products" (1554). Physicians' lack of knowledge about dietary supplements does indeed appear to be a primary factor in understanding why patients tend not to consult their physicians about them (Blendon et al.): if physicians do not know about the products patients want to take, patients will not ask about them. However, from the perspective of medical-professional boundary work, physicians' lack of knowledge about supplements only partly explains patients' reticence to discuss or disclose their use of supplements. There is also an interpersonal, interactive dimension to the problem.

The power dynamics of many practitioner-patient relationships, even strong ones, may leave patients worried about being judged or dismissed when disclosing their interest in dietary supplements. A 2001 study found, for example, that half of the respondents in national opinion surveys felt that doctors were "prejudiced against supplement use" (Blendon et al. 808). Further, the genre of the clinical consultation itself may not invite such off-script discussions: just as doctors tend to follow an unwritten code in their performance of the genre, so too do patients. While clinical communication is varied and dependent on many factors, including the purpose and context of the visit, consultations do follow familiar and generally predictable patterns. Within that communicative framework, the prospect of mentioning an interest in interventions that do not fit in that semiscripted environment may intimidate some patients. Additionally, given that many individuals view supplements as something that helps them maintain their health rather than to treat any specific illness (Nichter and Thompson), supplements may seem to be none of the doctor's business in the first place.

In his *JAMA* article, Mitka revisits the 1994 Dietary Supplement Health and Education Act (DSHEA), which redefined dietary supplements as akin to food products, not drugs (despite their often-profound pharmacologic effects). Unlike pharmaceutical legislation, which requires evidence of a product's safety and efficacy (however problematic that evidence may be), DSHEA rendered the FDA virtually toothless over products such as echinacea, bee pollen, and the now-banned ephedra, limiting its purview to investigation of aftermarket complaints of harm. DSHEA emerged out of an increasingly market-oriented approach to health care and its results have been far reaching, creating an ever freer health marketplace in which consumers are invited to buy better health in (typically) capsule form. Since 1994, biomedical stakeholders such as the American Medical Association have challenged that legislation but their arguments have not stood up well in the public arena: while biomedical discourse often sets the terms of debate in an increasingly medicalized society, dietary supplements—as readily available commercial products oriented to wellness, not illness—seem beyond medicine's reach.

Under DSHEA, dietary supplements can only make claims related to the structure or function of bodily systems but cannot make reference to disease. For example, a supplement can "support regularity" or "help maintain cardiovascular health" but not "alleviate constipation" or "lower cholesterol" (Mitka 1555). Structure-function claims limit how supplement producers may market their products, permitting only vague descriptions of their purposes and effects. Yet these kinds of claims do, at the same time, create an attractive discontinuity (in rhetorician Kenneth Burke's terms) between supplements' ostensible purpose, to *maintain wellness*, and that of pharmaceuticals, to *treat illness*. For example, if illness is the purview of biomedicine, then a product such as black cohosh, which "supports menopause," may well seem outside of that model. As Nichter and Thompson argue, this apparent discontinuity between drugs and supplements—and, by extension, between illness and wellness—contributes significantly to the prevalence of supplements in North America.

The rhetorical effects of such vague health claims turn out to be somewhat more complicated, however. On the one hand, Nichter and Thompson's study shows that these claims do give patients the sense that they are engaging in "harm reduction" (185) by substituting "toxic" pharmaceuticals with "natural" dietary supplements (192). And supplements do seem to support patients' wishes for "an increased sense of agency through an alternative diagnosis for their health concerns, additional treatment options, and a renewed sense of hope" (194). On the other hand, however, Nichter and Thompson also found that supplement users are savvy interpreters of structure-function claims, with many simply translating the products' wellness-oriented claims into illness-centered biomedical terms. For example, while a label might claim that black cohosh "supports menopause," users in their study simply made the cognitive leap from that generalized structure-function claim to the disease-symptom claim—that black cohosh will "reduce hot flashes."

Redefined under DSHEA as food-like substances, not drugs, dietary supplements have come to be seen by the public as more like eating one's vegetables than like taking drugs, despite their sometimes profound pharmacologic effects. Their use in combination with pharmaceuticals can result in drug interactions and other related morbidity (DeAngelis and Fontanarosa; Nisly et al.; Palmer et al.), and, in the case of hospitalized patients, serious complications and unexplained withdrawal effects can occur when supplement use is not reported. A letter in the *JAMA* theme issue outlines just such a case, of a fifty-eight-year-old man who, on admission to hospital, reported his regular medications—isosorbide dinitrate, digoxin, furosemide, benazepril, aspirin, lovastatin, ibuprofen, and multivitamins—but did not report concurrently taking between 530 mg and 2 g of valerian root five times per day (Garges, Varia, and Doraiswamy). As the patient's condition worsened, hospital staff were unaware that he was experiencing withdrawal. It was only when he experienced extreme pulmonary symptoms, tremulousness, and delirium that his family reported his use of valerian root to hospital staff, noting that he took it "to help him 'relax and sleep'" (1567).

Garges, Varia, and Doraiswamy conclude that physicians should be aware of the symptoms of valerian root withdrawal, since hospitals do not provide herbal preparations to inpatients. The authors contend that such potential problems could be avoided in the future by asking patients directly about their use of supplements. From both this scenario and the authors' proposed solution, a mandated communication script, we can pull several threads that illuminate further the role of practitioner-patient interaction in biomedical boundary work: that dietary supplements are perceived as "natural," and thus appear to be outside of biomedicine's purview; that clinical communication is central to discourses about supplements; and that access to supplements can for some patients translate into a sense of agency and autonomy. I explore these interrelated threads in closing.

By focusing on supplement safety, efficacy, and legislation, authors in the *JAMA-Archives* theme issues miss an important opportunity to query the reasons that lead so many individuals to favor unregulated, "natural" health interventions over more conventional and better-studied pharmaceuticals. For example, the reasons why someone would choose a herbal remedy such as St. John's wort over Prozac seems lost on many of the contributors in the *JAMA-Archives* theme issues, particularly since supplements function physiologically as if they are pharmaceuticals but lack the proof of efficacy that is the hallmark of evidence-based medicine. In the *JAMA-Archives*, authors such as Cirigliano and Sun and O'Hara et al. seek to dispel public misconceptions about herbal remedies and their pharmacological effects but they do not reflect on why individuals flock to dietary supplements even in the absence of an evidence base. Such reflection could yield important insight into how people perceive their own position as patients within health care contexts.

Dietary supplements hold an inherent persuasiveness that seems to promise users a significant sense of control over their health (Nichter and Thompson 189), inviting them to reimagine themselves as active agents of wellness, in Kenneth Burke's terms, rather than as passive scenes of illness (*Grammar* xv). Although supplements are usually sold as capsules or tablets, like pharmaceuticals, they otherwise seem antithetical: their packaging often features illustrations of leaves, flowers, or other symbols of nature, and earthy colors such as blue, green, and brown; they are often purchased in stores with wood floors and organic produce displays; and they are available without prescription, allowing consumers to decide for themselves what to take, how much, and how often. St. John's wort, for example, may be appealing to a depressed person whose condition has been thoroughly medicalized, whose physician has been unable to offer interpersonal support (due to lack of time or relevant training), and whose subsequent prescriptions for antidepressants have brought along with relief headache, nausea, dry mouth, weight gain, and the stigma of mental illness. Such individuals may prefer the herb's association with a small yellow flower (*Hypericum perforatum*) and a high internal locus of control over antidepressants' association with hugely profitable, impersonal pharmaceutical corporations and doctors who do not seem to care. In this light, the popularity of dietary supplements seems to stem, in part, from a desire for patients to regain control over their health within a medical system that this chapter has argued can be rhetorically disabling.

Judging from the prevalence of supplement use in the United States, members of the public clearly feel equipped to make their own decisions regarding dietary supplements. From a rhetorical perspective, however, we might question whether individuals really are prepared to make effective decisions about supplements within the discursive conditions of contemporary biomedicine. The precincts of care among different modalities of health, the generic features of practitioner-patient consultations, the argumentative weight of *evidence* in both the offering and making of choices, and the expanding geography of disease and illness—all of these conditions leave individuals considering dietary supplements in a double bind. Those who choose to consult with their doctors about supplements face a paucity of evidence and perhaps disapproval, while those who choose not to consult must negotiate an expanse of unverified and often conflicting information on the internet, in newspapers, magazines, and advertisements, and through salespeople and word of mouth.

A majority of commentators in the *JAMA-Archives* theme issues suggest that improved communication about CAM would better protect patients and even possibly stem the rising tide of individuals using or considering CAM. This may be true. But in the context of this book's larger argument about the ability of evidence to determine biomedical boundaries, we can more importantly view concerns about practitioner-patient interaction in debates about CAM as part of a larger constellation of concerns about the roles available to individuals in their own health care. Consumers' expanding demands for supplements under DSHEA's market-driven regulatory model lay bare tensions in biomedicine about patient agency and autonomy, and a rejection of impersonal, pharmaceutical-oriented health care. Dietary supplements have accrued such symbolic value, according to Kaptchuk and Eisenberg, that they "become daily activities of affirmation, assurance, and commitment. Dietary regimens . . . become liturgical acts of recognition with deeper implications for social, moral, and spiritual redemption" ("Persuasive" 1063; references removed). The symbolic value ascribed to supplement-taking as an act of self-empowerment is evident, for example, in protests against tighter supplement regulation, which I have examined elsewhere ("'Wellness'"). Such protests may be seen as largely about the rights of individuals, both as patients—recipients of medical interventions—and as consumers—choosers of interventions, from a menu of options. Further, if we consider that the notion of efficacy can be invoked to draw specific professional-epistemic boundary lines, then the question of whether or not a supplement "works" holds serious implications not only for the medical profession but also for individuals who seek supplements and the practitioners that treat them.

*

A key question that arises out of this chapter is through what means, and to what extent, patients can achieve autonomy over their own health care in an evidence-based framework. A rhetorical approach can open up some dimensions of this question in the context of biomedical research on CAM because it can demonstrate how the idea of "choice" may be framed within generic and rhetorical processes that tilt the course of decision-making in particular—and predictably biomedical—directions. It can also show, for example, how the idea of interaction itself can persuade in various directions: promises of more and better interaction with practitioners may persuade patients to seek chiropractors; a lack of control in clinical trials for interaction-related effects may persuade medical researchers not to take a trial's results seriously; and the desire to avoid interaction altogether may persuade individuals to choose dietary supplements over conventional pharmaceuticals.

The testing of interventions that depend significantly on interaction, such as those in CAM, opens health research up to practices and practitioners normally beyond the scope of conventional evidence frameworks, a movement that promises to humanize biomedicine's more positivist impulses. However, this wider scope of evidence production can also introduce new problems that hold far-reaching implications. For example, this wider scope threatens to expand biomedicine's authority through processes of surveillance and intervention. As sociologist Sam Porter cautions, "While the clinical gaze reduces us to our bodies, at least its surveillance is limited to those bodies. In contrast, by adding our psyche and our social circumstances to the gaze of health care workers, holistic care widens the trawl of surveillance to the most intimate parts of our lives" (19).

An expanded understanding of the myriad factors affecting health and illness is double-edged: it can enrich our knowledge of the things that make us sick and help us get well but can, at the same time, expand also the ways in which we *can* be sick, subsequently reformulating us increasingly as candidates for medical intervention. Put more simply, whatever their ameliorative potential, broader perspectives on health and illness have the potential, at the same time, to reinstall us anew within that same medicalizing system.

CAM practices such as acupuncture and chiropractic are brought into biomedicine's orbit as they are tested in clinical trials. Even biomedical interventions that are socially complex, such as nursing, are fundamentally transformed in research contexts as they are rendered amenable to quantification, isolation, and manipulation. And yet, although research on relational effects in health care poses significant challenges both to researchers and to practitioners attempting to integrate that research into practice, there are signs that biomedicine itself may be evolving through this expanded research program, as evidenced by the emergence of stratified models of placebo effects, which amplify and examine relationship effects within certain interventions rather than try to control for them.

This chapter has offered an account of how a thoroughly rhetorical activity—the clinical encounter—can irritate the notion of evidence and the markers of efficacy in medical interventions. It has argued that following the thread of practitioner-patient interaction through the landscape of testing CAM, as a set of socially complex interventions, can reflect something of the theoretical terrain of medicine itself. This process, in turn, lays the conceptual groundwork for further discussion of the ways that models of health research and practice circulate rhetorically, and how those models can shape the course of the practices, such as acupuncture and chiropractic, that they describe.

Professional Borders in Popular Media

"What is the real science of alternative medicine?" On December 2, 2002, *Newsweek* magazine posed this question in a special report called "Health for Life: Inside the Science of Alternative Medicine." Published as a mini-magazine within that week's regular issue, the special report locates the answer in the research on alternative medicine that emerged out of the 1998 founding of the National Center for Complementary and Alternative Medicine (NCCAM), the same year that the *Journal of the American Medical Association* (*JAMA*) and its related *Archives* specialty journals published the coordinated theme issues on complementary and alternative medicine (CAM). Although the *Newsweek* special report does not focus specifically on the *JAMA-Archives* theme issues, the magazine features numerous researchers whose work appeared within them. Prominently featured are David Eisenberg and Ted Kaptchuk, the Harvard medical school researchers who, following Eisenberg's major survey of Americans' CAM use and expenditure from 1993, led the charge to investigate alternative medicine in a biomedical framework. This issue of the magazine offers a comprehensive survey of research on CAM, from trial design to implementation of evidence to the larger implications of that research for medical professionals and the public. As with the *JAMA-Archives* theme issues, the *Newsweek* special report precipitated a wide-ranging response about research on CAM not only within biomedicine but also among CAM practitioners and within the wider public.

This final chapter of *Bounding Biomedicine* shifts us further downstream in the negotiation of biomedical boundaries, beyond the realm of practice into the public realm, to examine how evidence produced by studies of CAM is reported to nonspecialists. Focusing on the *Newsweek* special report,

I return to questions from earlier chapters regarding how texts surrounding scientific research on CAM, as discursive artifacts, negotiate medical-professional boundaries. Here, I examine the *Newsweek* report as a new set of interlinked texts, parallel to the *JAMA-Archives* theme issues, to examine how the magazine situates CAM and CAM research publicly vis-à-vis science as a bounded cultural space (Gieryn, *Cultural Boundaries*). As I have shown in previous chapters, even the most sincere biomedical investigations of alternative health practices are necessarily tilted against those practices, from acupuncture to yoga. The institutional-cultural forces that govern how such interventions are categorized and defined, tested experimentally, and implemented in practice do not blur boundaries between mainstream and alternative medicine as much as they reinforce and expand them. But what happens to those boundaries outside of research contexts? How are those boundaries configured when research on CAM is reported in the public realm? What values inhere in those reports—values about medical science and scientists; about mainstream medicine and alternative health modalities; and about ourselves, our bodies, and the ways that we understand and treat them?

To this point in the book, my rhetorical cartography of biomedicine has focused on texts and contexts that, if not fully internal to biomedicine, are still grounded in biomedical theory and practice. Practitioner-patient consultations, for example, occur fairly far downstream but nevertheless unfold in accordance with biomedical values and conventions. In this chapter, the texts I examine have a different set of allegiances, beyond the sphere of biomedicine. I investigate whether and how those texts work with, and within, biomedical terms. The intensive biomedical interest in CAM that began in the 1990s did not initially develop internally in medicine, in response to a problem identified by the medical profession as worthy of study. Instead, that interest came from outside, prompted by the public's unprecedented traffic toward CAM therapies and practitioners.

This is one of the reasons that the research reported in the *JAMA-Archives* theme issues proved controversial, because consumer behavior downstream, in everyday public life, appeared to have reverse-engineered behavior upstream, in medical research. For example, Angell and Kassirer lamented in their *New England Journal of Medicine* editorial published just two months prior to the *JAMA-Archives* theme issues that overwhelming but uncritical public interest in herbal remedies and other CAM therapies had forced the medical community to evaluate irrational and ineffective interventions that should have vanished long ago. Disparaging the research output of NCCAM's predecessor, the NIH Office of Alternative Medicine, as well as the legitimacy of the evidence it produced, Angell and Kassirer imply that well-meaning researchers had inappropriately reversed the lines of authority in science. By doing so, the editors seemed to be cautioning, the medical community had set a potentially dangerous precedent regarding how research priorities are set and by whom.

For members of the public, however, the scientific testing of CAM signaled a positive shift along the boundary between mainstream and alternative medicine. The tone of the *Newsweek* special report was celebratory as it praised medicine for finally responding to the growing public interest in practices that do not fit the standard scientific model of illness and health. The powerful medical profession appeared to have softened, taking seriously practices it had once dismissed. *Newsweek* praised the new research as "revolutionizing clinical practice and giving birth to a new kind of integrative medicine" ("Special Report" 45).

In her study of representations of science in print media of the first half of the twentieth century, historian Marcel LaFollette argues that "mass circulation magazines serve as especially sensitive indicators of what their readers believed (or wanted to believe) about science" (20). Sociologist Dorothy Nelkin similarly suggests that scientific reporting "reflects current fashions and editorial perceptions of what readers want to hear" about science (45). Such a view of public representations of science as barometers of what the public both believes and wants to believe about science highlights the reciprocal, rather than unidirectional, nature of science reporting. Consideration of this reciprocity between science and its publics draws renewed attention toward the classical rhetorical notion of audience: audiences help to determine how science is reported. In what follows, I foreground the reciprocity between speakers and listeners in popular reporting on science by suggesting that, more than merely reflecting what the public wants to believe about science, news coverage of CAM research shows how ideas about biomedicine and its boundaries circulate, in all directions, in popular contexts—ideas about how biomedicine operates; about the quantity and quality of the knowledge that it produces; about its potential costs, benefits, and risks; and about its agents and its consumers.

The movement of this book in the negotiation of biomedical boundaries from upstream contexts to down- is not an argument from arrangement, either about the relative priority of any one position along the spectrum of science or about the directions of influence among them. Rather, as science and technology studies scholar Stephen Hilgartner explains, the scope of texts and contexts that can properly be called "scientific" is wide and the point at which "science" becomes "popular science"—and so, by implication, not really "science" at all—is blurry, context-dependent, and "a matter of degree.

The boundary between real science and popularized science can be drawn at various points depending on what criteria one adopts" (528). I close my book with this final chapter on popular reporting about biomedical research on CAM not, then, because such reporting is the last stop on our journey along the boundary between mainstream and alternative medicine, but because it marks a point of recirculation: the chapter marks the return of CAM, filtered through science, to the public that motivated the research. In the texts at the center of this chapter, the nature of that return is my object of focus.

Studies of popular science have themselves contributed to the reification of boundaries between popular science and science proper. Jeanne Fahnestock's seminal 1986 article "Accommodating Science: The Rhetorical Life of Scientific Facts" was not the first to adopt what has since been critiqued as the "dominant model" of popularization (Hilgartner) but it exemplifies that model.[1] Fahnestock argues that accommodations (or translations) of science are "primarily epideictic"—"their main purpose is to celebrate rather than validate" ("Accommodating" 333). Fahnestock's framework presupposes a knowledge deficit in which scientific knowledge is interpreted by science reporters for the lay public. These reporters adapt "new knowledge to old assumptions and [try] to bridge the enormous gap between the public's right to know and the public's ability to understand" ("Accommodating" 331). In other words, according to Fahnestock, scientific information travels one way, from knowledgeable experts to an ignorant public. Later scholars such as Hilgartner and Alan Gross have argued vehemently against this unidirectional model, while Greg Myers emphasizes the range of possibilities between the poles of "expert" and "lay" in discourses on science. Myers critiques studies that, like Fahnestock's, trace research articles to their appearance in popular venues, an activity that he argues maintains the "dominant" view of popular science as simply handmaiden to science.

As Gross, Hilgartner, and Myers each show, popular science does not simply spread the word of science to the laity, reporting on its marvels and lamenting its missteps. On the contrary, as Gieryn argues, science's pride of place in contemporary Western culture is explicitly authorized by the very public that prizes it. Gieryn entreats us, therefore, to examine science not upstream through the construction of facts but downstream, where those facts circulate in the larger culture, because this is where science and scientists accrue their power to make and remake facts about the natural world. Something within downstream science itself must therefore contribute to the authority of science as it weighs in on an increasingly wide range of issues affecting human life.

Downstream science is not simply complicit in maintaining science's cultural dominance, however. Rather, I share with Danette Paul the view that popular science feeds back into the disciplines whose research it popularizes, not just describing science as it is but shaping how it will be. By viewing popular audiences as more than simply "ignorant and dependent" (Bensaude-Vincent 101), we may begin to see real consequences for science in even unambiguously popular texts, such as mass-circulation newspapers and magazines.[2]

One of my overarching arguments in this chapter is that medical reporting is a special case of science reporting, that it is both typical and exceptional. It is typical because medicine's research values, professional practices, generic forms, and institutional structures are closely aligned with those of science, yet it is exceptional because popular reporting on medicine can influence publicly held attitudes toward health and illness, which can, in turn, shape individual health beliefs and behaviors. This is not to say that popular readers necessarily find reports on health and medicine more important or more interesting than they do those on science; indeed, for many readers, popular reporting on health may hit a little too close to home, with the volume and evolving nature of its content overwhelming. (Foods we are impelled to eat one day for their nutrient content, for example, are disparaged the next, and then praised again following that. . . .)

My argument is instead that we, collectively, get a sense of what the stories about health in public circulation are, and that they affect us, even if, individually, we do not read those stories ourselves. I am borrowing here on Judy Segal's discussion in *Health and the Rhetoric of Medicine* of Mary McCarthy's novel, *The Group*. In the novel, a doctor tells the daughter of his patient, "We've noticed that now that we no longer speak of dementia praecox, we get fewer dementia-praecox patients. It tempts you to think sometimes that all mental illness has a hysterical origin, that they're all copying the latest textbooks. Even the illiterate patients" (qtd. in Segal 80). As Segal argues, stories in public circulation about health (and, I would add, about research on health), can effectively re-story us and how we think about ourselves as bodies, as patients, as people. So, while reporting on the latest in medical research may take on the same appearance and tone as reporting on the latest research in, say, particle physics, its rhetorical functions are importantly different because the stories that circulate in public about health and medicine can make us into different sorts of people.[3]

In making this distinction between the rhetoric of popular science and popular medicine, I am not arguing along the lines of what Miriam Solomon identifies as the "medicine is 'not a science,' or 'not only a science'" cliché common to discussions about the humanities and medicine, narrative and

medicine, or ethics and medicine (406). While the cliché that Solomon examines centers on the epistemology of medicine itself—whether or not medicine is a science—the split I am postulating here is instead about whether or
not *popular* medicine is best thought of, from the perspective of rhetoric, as
simply a variety of *popular* science. I think we can answer the second question
without considering the first.

The first section of the chapter examines the *Newsweek* special report as
a significant rhetorical moment in the production and maintenance of biomedical boundaries, on the order of the *JAMA-Archives* theme issues. The
second and third sections take up popular medicine as a typical case in popular science. The second section explicates the model of the "new science" of
CAM introduced in *Newsweek*. Despite the magazine's claims about the novelty and scope of this new model, the magazine turns out to offer a fairly
standard story of science and scientific research. In the third section, I trace
how CAM is situated vis-à-vis that standard model of science by examining
a recurrent rhetorical construction in the special report that asks of CAM,
"Does it really work?" Both of these sections are concerned with medicine as
it is installed within scientific modes of thinking and practice, and with the
ways in which CAM is variously lined up with them.

The remaining sections take up popular medicine as an exceptional case in
popular science. The fourth section begins with questions of expertise in medicine, using the magazine's clear differentiation between biomedical experts
and nonexperts to find where, and how, the magazine establishes boundaries
between scientific professionals and the lay public. The final, fifth section pulls
together the various narratives about CAM that underlie the *Newsweek* report,
collected over the course of the chapter, to examine what they do *not* tell us.
The stories that the magazine does not tell about both CAM and biomedicine
can point to potential problems as biomedicine's boundaries shift, expanding
to increasing areas of human life. Science studies scholars such as Gieryn and
Felicity Mellor suggest that downstream science plays a significant part in the
production and maintenance of science's cultural and epistemic authority; the
work of this chapter, accordingly, sheds important light on the public processes through which some health practices come to count in contemporary
biomedicine as legitimate and others, not.

The *Newsweek* Special Report as a Biomedical "Discourse Moment"

The *Newsweek* special report served as a flashpoint of debate about the boundaries between mainstream and alternative medicine. At the time of its publication, *Newsweek* had the second-highest paid circulation in its category next

to *Time* (3.2 million versus 4.1 million), and was ranked nineteenth overall in American magazines (Magazine Publishers of America). When the special report hit newsstands in late 2002, debate spread quickly both in academic and popular media, especially in the blogosphere. Robert Park, for instance, a University of Maryland physicist and author of *Voodoo Science: The Road from Foolishness to Fraud*, featured *Newsweek* on his weekly online newsletter to draw firm boundaries about what he believed ought to count as proper to medical science. Park writes: "The cover story in the Dec 2 issue of Newsweek is The Science of Alternative Medicine. That's an oxymoron. If these alternatives had a basis in science, they would just be medicine. *Newsweek* calls it 'The New Science.'" Similarly, both the National Council Against Health Fraud's monthly newsletter and the consumer website *Quackwatch* devoted significant space to denouncing the *Newsweek* special report, methodically detailing twenty-one "problems" associated with the magazine's treatment of what they call "sCAM" ("so-called Complementary and Alternative Medicine"; London).

The *Newsweek* special report also ignited intense excitement among CAM practitioners. CAM-professional news websites such as *Acupuncture Today*, *Dynamic Chiropractic*, and *Massage Today*, collectively published by the alternative-medical organization MPA Media, offered uniformly positive assessments of the magazine.[4] However, not all CAM practitioners saw the special report as an unequivocal good. For example, in communication researcher Evelyn Ho's ethnographic study of student acupuncturists, the magazine's publication precipitated what she characterizes as a "social drama," a pattern of discursive activity produced in response to a perceived violation of social norms (421). This social drama was so significant among her study's participants that she situated their response to the *Newsweek* report as the focal point of her larger project on speech codes at the study site, an acupuncture training clinic. These examples of the public response to the *Newsweek* special report collectively attest to its importance in debates about biomedical research on CAM, illustrating in turn the magazine's significance as a site of rhetorical boundary work in popular media.

As a textual artifact, the *Newsweek* special report mirrors the *JAMA-Archives* theme issues. It, too, is a multilayered, bounded discursive object, a self-contained version of what Sophie Moirand calls a "discourse moment" in science popularization, a "surge of intense and diversified media activity in connection with a single media event" (178)—in this case, the highly publicized boom of CAM research beginning around 1998. The report spans a considerable range of the genres, topics, and authorial expertise that constitute medical reporting: from sidebars offering explicit medical advice to complex, long-form explorations of a given specialty's state-of-the-art; from deadly diseases to chronic and mental illness to health maintenance; from care of the young to that of the old; with articles by nonspecialist reporters, seasoned medical journalists, and expert medical researchers and practitioners. The *Newsweek* special report does not cover all possible varieties of popular medicine (it does not feature, for example, sustained first-person accounts of illness) but it does provide a rich cross-section of the different kinds of medical reporting available among the popular media, presented together as a dossier on the "new science" of CAM.

Unlike single popular articles across disparate publications, these articles are meant, like those of a dossier, to be read together. The ways in which they can be read with and against one another are important from a rhetorical standpoint because they permit us to examine layered trajectories of persuasion within a multidimensional whole—in individual articles, across articles and sections, and among and across different sorts of authors. The report itself is structured as a magazine-within-a-magazine, with its own title page and table of contents in the middle section of the magazine. It is divided into three separate sections, each section with two feature articles, other short articles, sidebars, and related infographics. The sections are interlinked by their common visual format, with a shared graphic design unique to the report, and by a recurring sidebar feature, "Insights from Harvard Medical School," that appears throughout on topics such as osteoarthritis, cancer, and "research."

The texts within each of the three sections are themselves interwoven in both theme and layout, with some articles set inside and around others, and all sharing common section headers. The first section, "The New Science," opens with the article "Now, 'Integrative' Care" (Cowley), which doubles as the lead article of the whole special report. This article, twice the length of the next-longest articles, sets the stage for what follows by surveying the current state of research on, institutional and regulatory support for, and patient use of complementary and alternative medicine. The article "Learning from China" (Underwood) follows, exploring the potential contributions of traditional Chinese medicine to biomedicine. The second major section, "Family Health," looks at alternative medicine for children (Noonan, "For the Littlest Patients") and for women (Kalb, "A Natural Way to Age"); and the third section explores "Mind and Moods," covering anxiety and depression (Kalb, "How to Lift the Mind") and placebo effects (Kaptchuk, Eisenberg, and Komaroff, "Pondering the Placebo Effect"). Each of these sections features sidebars and infographics that take up the topics discussed in the articles themselves; I describe these sidebars and infographics below. All of the articles in the special report are presented as an integrated set of cotexts—curated, as it were, to present a cohesive statement on the "new science" of CAM—and so they can provide important meta-level insight into how that new science is constructed within the public realm.[5]

In the service of my larger study, the *Newsweek* report is a useful counterpoint to the *JAMA-Archives* theme issues. Both sets of texts share a concerted focus on CAM as an area of scientific inquiry and each covers a wide range of health conditions and CAM practices. Throughout this book, I have argued that the *JAMA-Archives* theme issues can be read as an artifact of a specific rhetorical moment as the American Medical Association stakes a claim, through its publication arm, in the debate surrounding complementary and alternative medicine. We can similarly read the *Newsweek* special report as a rhetorical artifact, but one with a quite different orientation. Unlike *JAMA* and the *Archives*, whose examination of CAM ultimately serves the interests of medical researchers and practitioners as a defined professional community, *Newsweek* offers a complex meditation on biomedical boundary work that aims to meet the conflicting interests of its various stakeholders, including advertisers, editors, journalist-authors, researcher-authors, and general and expert readers. The picture of the "new science" offered across the articles is therefore multilayered; by tracking these layers across articles by different authors and on different subjects within a cohesive "discourse moment," we can learn more about the variability of rhetorical boundaries in biomedicine.

Reporting the New Science

In answer to the *Newsweek* special report's key question, "What is the real science of alternative medicine?" the magazine makes the case that a fundamentally new model of science had emerged over recent years, one that was premised on open-minded assessment of health practices that medical researchers and practitioners had long dismissed as superstitious quackery. This new model appeared seamlessly to integrate multiple modalities into a single, scientific whole. As Geoffrey Cowley noted in his lead article, "At many of the country's leading hospitals and research institutions, conventionally trained physicians are studying herbs, acupuncture, tai chi and biofeedback as rigorously as they would a new antibiotic" (48). Applying scientific methods to centuries-old traditions, Cowley argued, these physician-researchers were on the cusp of producing a "new blend of medicine" (47), an equal merging of mainstream and alternative treatments that would revolutionize health care and health research.

Of course, this new, blended "science" of CAM likely held no special appeal to the millions of Americans already enthusiastic about nonmainstream health practices. More importantly, what appears in the magazine at first to be a radical new vision of scientific medicine as dynamic and inclusive was ultimately not particularly new, nor was it inclusive. Even still, tracking the magazine's discursive construction of an ostensibly new, scientific model of CAM can usefully illustrate something of what the public believes (or wants to believe) about biomedicine. In turn, such analysis can illuminate the means through which ideas (and ideals) about biomedical boundaries circulate in public. As Bradley Lewis notes in his study of a 2001 *Newsweek* special report on biotechnology, "Only through studying artifacts like *Newsweek* can medical humanities scholars uncover the contemporary cultural and political dimensions of biomedicine" (365). To articulate some of these dimensions vis-à-vis biomedical boundary work, I offer a close reading of the *Newsweek* special report on CAM in this section and the one that follows.

Over the *Newsweek* report's pages, we learn three principal things about the "science of alternative medicine," which together produce a conflicted account of how complementary and alternative medicine fit within a biomedical framework. The first thing we learn is that such a science exists, and everything within the *Newsweek* report seems orchestrated to provide evidence of that epistemic claim. For instance, the report's opening question—"What is the real science of alternative medicine?"—presupposes linguistically the prior existence of a real, known entity, a *science of alternative medicine*.[6] The question also simultaneously presupposes a separate category, a *not-real science of alternative medicine*, a pseudoscientific CAM, perhaps, or just an indifferently unscientific one. However we might imagine this not-real science of CAM, the key point here is that the question itself, "What is the real science of alternative medicine?" invites us to make distinctions among different kinds of CAM, from what the magazine defines as "credible" (acupuncture, chiropractic, herbal therapies) to the "laughable" (coffee enemas; 48). Only the first kind of CAM, the credible, is genuinely scientific in the magazine's view, and the special report poises itself to tell more about only that.

The magazine makes similar declarations about the science of CAM throughout the special report, each inflecting different binaries akin to the binary of "real" and "not-real." The subtitle of the report, for example, promises to take us "*Inside* the Science of Alternative Medicine" (45; emphasis added), casting the science of CAM in spatially exclusive terms of inside and outside. Here, "the science of alternative medicine" is designated as unfamiliar territory, a bounded space into which we, as outsiders, need to be guided by the magazine. Drawing boundaries of a different sort, the title of the first of the magazine's three major sections, "The New Science," distinguishes between old and new. For being new, the science of CAM is unlike any extant variety or model of science, and is therefore individually identifiable as *the* new science, not merely *a* new science or *one of the* new sciences.

Perhaps more importantly, this new science is specifically geared for alternative medicine, as if it were a custom-made form of science. In all of these binary constructions—real/not-real, inside/outside, new/old—the science of alternative medicine is constructed, above all, as appreciably different from the science we have known before: it is a science transformed.

The first thing we learn in *Newsweek*, then, is that there is a (new) science of CAM. The second thing we learn is that this new science is *integrative*, based on the resolution of several sets of oppositions: alternative and mainstream, old and new, East and West, and care and cure. In the broader culture, as CAM has come into the mainstream over recent decades, claims to integration have played a key role in its persuasive force. For instance, naturopaths in the Canadian provinces of British Columbia and Ontario now have pharmaceutical prescribing rights, integrating pharmacological interventions into their multimodal, nature-centric practice, while my local hospital in Toronto offers acupuncture among its suite of adjuvant therapies in a multidisciplinary treatment center for arthritis and autoimmune disease. Integration between biomedicine and CAM flows both ways, appearing to offer the benefits of multiple modalities in a single framework, although as I have suggested in earlier chapters, that flow is seldom free or even. For the magazine, however, the notion of integration is central to its thesis that the new science of alternative medicine represents a revolution in American health care.

One of the *Newsweek* report's primary means of persuasion about the integrative quality of this new science of CAM is its visual composition. The magazine constructs a "visual metonymy," in Russell Willerton's terms, that illustrates graphically the union of mainstream and alternative medicine and all of their embedded sets of oppositions (alternative/mainstream, old/new, East/West, care/cure.) Examining "stage-setting images" in technical communication, Willerton bases his concept of visual metonymy on Karen Schriver's model of document design, which in turn expands I. A. Richards's concept of interanimation from linguistic contexts to the reciprocal influence of words and images. Drawing on Schriver's work, Willerton defines stage-setting images as those that develop and support, or *interanimate*, themes advanced in written texts (4). He argues that stage-setting images often perform the "distilling functions of synecdoche and metonymy" by depicting "tangible" aspects of a given theme (11), such as the image of a gavel as visually metonymic of the law (his example). Such tangible, stage-setting images, he argues, convey thematic content by inducing readers to make specific associations related to that theme.

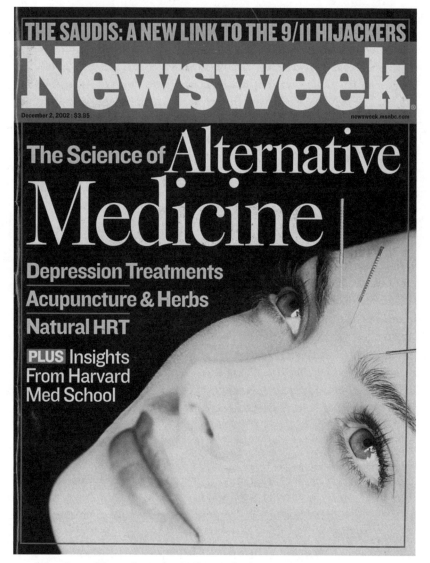

THE SAUDIS: A NEW LINK TO THE 9/II HIJACKERS

Newsweek

December 2, 2002 : $3.95   newsweek.msnbc.com

The Science of Alternative

Medicine

Depression Treatments

Acupuncture & Herbs

Natural HRT

PLUS Insights
From Harvard
Med School

FIGURE 3. Cover of *Newsweek* magazine: Wolfgang Ludes, *Newsweek* 2 Dec. 2002.

In the *Newsweek* report, visual metonymy sets up patterns of association that develop the theoretical concept of integration through the depiction of "tangibles," such as health practitioners and patients, in settings that include elements of both the mainstream and the alternative. The cover, for instance, features a tight shot of a woman's face against a flat black backdrop (see fig. 3). The woman, smiling serenely with open, upward-facing eyes and three acupuncture needles placed just above and between her eyebrows, seems to be of European origin and does not look like a person we might associate with a particular subculture. This seems exactly to be the point: the photo is at once familiar and exotic, mundane and sensational. Generic, tranquil, and punctured by steel needles, this woman embodies both literally and metaphorically the fusion of binaries that characterize the "new science" as it is depicted in *Newsweek*.

The cover text both contains and constrains this characterization of the new science as integrative. The main cover line, "The Science of Alternative Medicine," sets up a relational dynamic between the three terms *science, alternative,* and *medicine,* with "Alternative" about double the size of "The Science of" and "Medicine" at least triple that size.[7] The difference in font size indicates a hierarchical relationship between medicine and its adjective: the needles in the woman's face may be alternative but they are, more significantly, medicine. This emphasis on medicine as an authorizing entity is further reinforced underneath the main cover line and the three smaller-font cover lines advertising the report's feature articles on depression treatments, acupuncture and herbal medicine, and natural hormone replacement, as well as a bonus ("PLUS") of "Insights from Harvard Med School." This invocation of Harvard creates a strong association between the potentially sensational image of the woman with the needles in her face and one of the United States' most prestigious medical schools, as if to say, "Not only is this needle-based practice medicine, it's Harvard-approved."

Similar visual patterns linking ideas of alternative and mainstream, old and new, East and West, and care and cure are found throughout the magazine. For example, the initial facing pages of Geoffrey Cowley's lead article, "Now, 'Integrative' Care," features a full-color photograph spanning three-quarters of the spread, depicting radiologist Zang-Hee Cho and a colleague, both clearly of Asian descent, performing acupuncture on a patient's bare feet in a biomedical setting (see fig. 4). Both men wear white lab coats while their patient lies inside a prominently pictured functional magnetic resonance imaging (fMRI) machine. The article's title, superimposed on the photo, makes a claim that, given the strong visual associations within the photo itself, seems almost superfluous: "Now, 'Integrative' Care." As readers, we bring to the image assumptions triggered by the image's metonymic content that make the case for the integration of medical models before we even read the article itself: lab coats and fMRI machines represent biomedicine; acupuncture needles represent alternative medicine; their copresence represents *integration*. Through these images, we come to the text primed to hear more about "The New Science" of integrative care because we have already seen visual evidence of it in action. And so, when Cowley claims in the text of the article that the

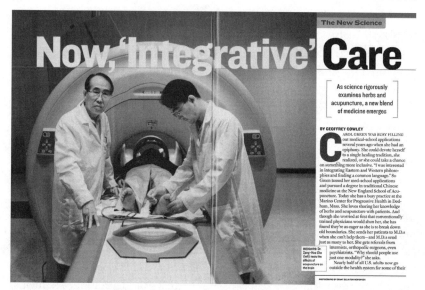

FIGURE 4. "INSIGHTS: Dr Zang-Hee Cho (left) Tests the Effects of Acupuncture on the Brain," Grant Delin, *Newsweek* 2 Dec. 2002: 46–47.

main goal of CAM research is "to spawn a new kind of medicine—an *integrative* medicine that employs the rigor of modern science [to create] one health system instead of two" (48), the claim may not seem like news to us.

Other photographs in the report support this claim to integration, particularly when the images are read against their surrounding text. For example, the second set of facing pages in Cowley's article stand in stark contrast to the article itself: while the text reports on institutional research culture, political wrangling, and government funding, the accompanying photographs depict patients engaging in behaviors that one would not normally associate with institutionalized medicine. One holds a yoga pose on a wood floor, wearing a vibrant green silk shirt and black leggings (importantly, not a paper gown; see fig. 5); the other, an inpatient, wears her own clothes while lying on a bed with a plaid and floral bedspread, singing along with a woman playing guitar (see fig. 6). The pairing of these images and text evokes a sense of balance among oppositions, such as institutional/individual, impersonal/personal, mainstream/alternative, and even cure/care. Such balance is crucial to activity that could fairly be called "integrative." Similarly, Claudia Kalb's "A Natural Way to Age" focuses on the state of medical research on treatments for menopause, but the photos depict everyday women in nonmedical settings: one stands smiling, in a pumpkin patch with her family, while the other stands, midlaugh, at a hot dog stand. Both women seem relaxed and happy in spite of their menopause, as if to affirm that integrative medicine works.

The text that accompanies these images similarly frames the new integrative medicine as the product of an enthusiastic and equal marriage between science and practices such as acupuncture and herbal medicine. Science and alternative medicine appear to balance each other. Cowley's lead article

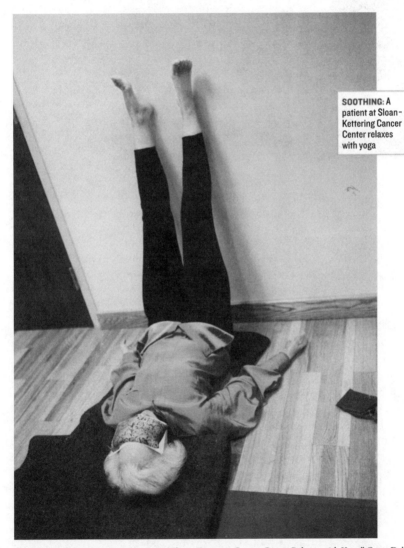

SOOTHING: A patient at Sloan-Kettering Cancer Center relaxes with yoga

FIGURE 5. "SOOTHING: A Patient at Sloan-Kettering Cancer Center Relaxes with Yoga," Grant Delin, *Newsweek* 2 Dec. 2002: 48.

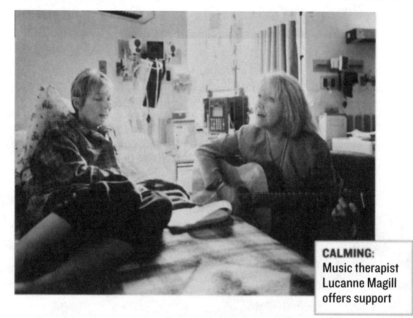

CALMING:
Music therapist
Lucanne Magill
offers support

FIGURE 6. "CALMING: Music Therapist Lucanne Magill Offers Support," Grant Delin, *Newsweek* 2 Dec. 2002: 49.

makes the strongest claims about integration, particularly in his opening with the story of Carol Green's "epiphany" while applying to medical school. Realizing that she wanted to explore a more "inclusive" mode of health care,

> Green tossed her med-school applications and pursued a degree in traditional Chinese medicine at the New England School of Acupuncture. Today she has a busy practice [and]. . . . though she worried at first that conventionally trained physicians would shun her, she has found they're as eager as she is to break down old boundaries. She sends her patients to MDs when she can't help them—and MDs send just as many to her. She gets referrals from internists, orthopedic surgeons, even psychiatrists. "Why should people use just one modality?" she asks. (47)

In this case, balance among binaries is represented in the professional activity of referral, a reciprocity that implies that TCM and biomedicine share a friendly, undefended border. The assumption here is that plurality is good, a perspective that ultimately does not mesh with scientific empiricism and the place it accords to evidence in medical decision-making, but one that gives us a window into public attitudes about health and illness, particularly within frameworks of consumer choice.

Similar claims about successful biomedical-alternative integration are made throughout the *Newsweek* report, all offering positive accounts about the new science of CAM. In David Noonan's article about kids and CAM, we hear about twelve-year-old Christie Blackwood, who was referred to the Minneapolis Children's Hospital Department of Integrative Medicine and Cultural Care after a week of struggling with the side effects of chemotherapy for leukemia. Christie was taught about acupressure, biofeedback, aromatherapy, and guided imagery, the last of which, her mother reports, kept Christie from vomiting even once, despite vomiting severely with chemotherapy alone. Noonan writes that kids are "the most important ingredient" in integrative pediatric care—"Like Christie Blackwood, calm and cheerful in the face of cancer, combining the power of chemotherapy and the power of her imagination as she wages the fight of her life" (62). The marriage of biomedicine and CAM has given Christie agency over her treatment where, we might assume, she would have otherwise had none.

The medical director of Christie's clinic, Timothy Culbert, tells Noonan that, among primary-care pediatricians, "CAM is on the tip of everybody's tongue every day" (59). This statement, though undoubtedly true for Culbert and other physicians working in specialty integrative medicine clinics, does not fully capture the position of most practicing American doctors, then or now, who remain largely ambivalent, if open-minded, about the clinical effects of complementary and alternative medicine. Certainly, Cowley and Underwood's similar claim in a 1998 *Newsweek* article about the *JAMA-Archives* theme issues, that "*JAMA*'s editors are now accepting yoga and acupuncture as facts of life" (68), could not withstand scrutiny. Although many individuals find great benefit in each practice, the medical literature is short on clear evidence of their effectiveness. Furthermore, as I have argued in earlier chapters, when there is strong evidence of a CAM intervention's effect, questions remain for many medical researchers and practitioners about causality—does acupuncture work by stimulating energy flow (a traditional Chinese medicine explanation) or by stimulating the release of endorphins (a biomedical explanation), or are its effects produced instead by patient expectation (placebo effects)?

These articles offer accounts of integration that seem more to reflect the ideals of *Newsweek*'s readership than the current state of American medicine. Consider again Cowley's opening story of Carol Green, who, after "toss[ing] her med-school applications," studied traditional Chinese medicine and then took up work at the Marino Center for Progressive Health in Dedham, MA. What Cowley does not make clear in his article is that the Marino Center is a specialty integrative medicine clinic, and that the referrals that Green makes to and from MDs may be internal among her colleagues at the clinic. In making assertions such as this about the extent and success of integration in the new science of alternative medicine, *Newsweek* overstates the level of reciprocity among biomedical and alternative practices and practitioners.

In the public sphere, however, science is not a monolithic, authorizing authority; it is simply one way of knowing among many. The label of "science" does hold significant cultural weight, as evidenced in the grafting of the term as a suffix onto other academic disciplines (political science, social science, computer science), religions (Christian science, Scientology), and even consumer products (Earth Science cosmetics, Science Diet pet foods).[8] In public culture, by contrast, views of science are frequently tempered with skepticism and scientists are often viewed as blinkered by scientific dogma. In this light, the magazine's assertion that integrative care is already an accepted fact of medical life in the United States suggests more about the values and interests of *Newsweek*'s readers, and about their desire to pick and choose among health care modalities, than it does about how mainstream scientific medicine operates.

The first thing we learn in the *Newsweek* special report, then, is that there exists a brand-new science of CAM—one that we learn, second, is integrative. But we learn a third thing in the magazine too, which ultimately supersedes the first two: what is lauded in the magazine as a new, integrative medical science is, in substance, neither new nor integrative. While it is true that biomedicine is depicted in *Newsweek* as vulnerable to boundary incursion, with researchers "racing" to catch up to the demands of the CAM-interested public (Cowley 48), the fundamental nature of biomedicine itself—its ways of knowing, its modes of care—remains essentially unchanged. In fact, although the magazine praises biomedicine for opening up its borders to unconventional health care, those borders do not appear in the magazine as open and permeable but as expanded and fortified. Much as I argued in chapter 1 about the *JAMA* and *Archives* theme issues, the *Newsweek* special report situates biomedicine as the final arbiter of whether or not alternative medical practices such as acupuncture and herbal remedies are deemed safe and effective. That sort of medicine is imperial, not integrative.

The idea of integrative medicine has long held an appeal in the popular media. In 1993, nearly ten years prior to the *Newsweek* special report, Sharon Begley and Debra Rosenberg argued, also in *Newsweek*, that Americans were "clamoring for alternatives to drugs, surgery and doctors who treat them as nothing but bags of symptoms" (61). The answer, for these alternative-seeking individuals, seemed to have been found in integrative medicine. As physicians

Wendy Weiger and David Eisenberg explain in the 2002 special report, "Unlike conventional treatments, which can leave a person feeling passive and helpless, many complementary therapies help patients become active participants in their care" (49). Patients under this new model are no longer mere "bags of symptoms," argue Weiger and Eisenberg, but are instead empowered and valued. Similar such statements are found throughout the special report but their accumulation does not ultimately advance a claim to "integration" between mainstream and alternative medicine as much as these statements highlight the incongruity of the claim itself within the conventional model of science that underlies the report.

Consider again the photos in the Cowley and Kalb articles I describe above: while they do set the stage for claims such as Cowley's that "Doctors are as unhappy as patients about the current state of health care, and most are eager to make it more caring and humane" (48), evaluated more closely, the patients in these pictures seem superfluous to the drama that unfolds around them. On the first page of Cowley's article, for example, all we can see of Dr. Cho's acupuncture patient are his or her bare feet and clothed body; the rest is obscured inside the fMRI machine (fig. 4). And while we do see patients' whole bodies in the article's other photos, their captions direct our attention toward the modes of treatment rather than those being treated: "A patient at Sloan-Kettering Cancer Center relaxes with yoga" (48; fig. 5); "Music therapist Lucanne Magill offers support" (49; fig. 6). In the first caption, the clinic is identified by name (Sloan-Kettering Cancer Center) but not the patient, whose face is covered with a small sachet. The focus in the second caption is the therapist, not the patient, even though both are equally visible. The anonymity of the women in these images renders them iconic, and therefore may help readers to identify more closely with them. But for that same reason, the women themselves, as individuals, retreat from view. The individualized care associated with CAM becomes somewhat standardized in these images, with the women standing in as generic patients, the spotlight not on them but on their treatment in a hospital setting.

The women depicted in Kalb's article about menopause treatments seem no more three-dimensional even though they do have names. In fact, whereas the photographs in the Cowley article seem like stock images of patients in CAM settings, the women in Kalb's article seem not only generic but, depicted in a pumpkin patch and at hot dog stand respectively, comparatively insignificant when set against Kalb's narrative of the sprawling institutional and regulatory fallout of the hormone replacement therapy scandal.

The idea of integration, the blending of mainstream and alternative medicine, is likewise elusive in the accompanying articles. Cowley's lead article sets up the special report's key claim that a "new blend of medicine" has be-gun to emerge (47), one that will "employ . . . the rigor of modern science without being constrained by it" (48), but this claim founders even over the course of his own article. Only paragraphs after describing the new science as a "blend," Cowley asks: "Can a system built on one paradigm accommo-date another? Is there room for care and compassion within science-based medicine?" (50). What he describes here is not two systems merging into one, as he first claims, but, rather, one system (biomedicine) absorbing another (alternative medicine). The distinction between merging and absorbing may be subtle, but it captures the directional flow of knowledge and power in the context of scientific research on alternative medicine, a flow that maintains hierarchies rather than effaces them.

As I have argued in previous chapters, the constraining force of "rigor" is precisely what makes science culturally recognizable as science, so it is no wonder that what is packaged throughout the *Newsweek* special report as "in-tegrative" turns out instead to be tilted unambiguously toward biomedicine. Whether it is Underwood describing "cutting-edge research" on acupunc-ture points, now linked not to energy meridians but to thickness of connec-tive tissue ("Learning" 56), or Kalb framing menopause-related discomfort as symptoms of biological dysfunction, biomedical science retains executive powers in its ostensible marriage with CAM: it holds sole authority to deter-mine whether or not a CAM practice works. What I argue next is that the distance between the new, integrative science of CAM that *Newsweek* claims to report on and the conventionally scientific model that actually undergirds the special report brings into focus some of the tensions that underlie popular reporting on science and medicine. The model of science advanced in the special report is more complex than the literature on rhetorics of popular sci-ence would suggest, and, for that complexity, its boundaries are both broader and stronger.

"Does it Really Work?" Constructing Biomedicine in the Media

In the *Newsweek* special report, the science of complementary and alterna-tive medicine has two faces. One face is outward-looking and authoritative, an objective, methodical science able to adjudicate confidently on matters of human health and health care. It is what Latour calls a "ready-made" science (13), centered on the principle of consensus within communities of scientists. But the other face of *Newsweek*'s science of CAM is more anxious and uncer-tain: inward-looking, it is marked by disagreement rather than consensus; in Latour's terms, it is a science "in the making" (13). While ready-made science takes current available knowledge as solid enough grounds to decide future courses of action, for science-in-the-making, there are always further questions to be asked and further answers to be sought.

The intellectual labor of upstream science (in laboratories, conferences, and peer-reviewed publications) tends toward science-in-the-making, predicated on ever-receding standards of what counts as sufficient evidence of or against a scientific claim. Downstream science (in public policy and popular media) instead tends toward science as ready-made: with each new study, we know more and are able to do more with that knowledge. The *Newsweek* special report is unusual as an instance of popular reporting on science because, rather than tending toward the ready-made, as popular science typically does, the magazine equivocates between the two faces of science.[9]

In this section, I argue that, through the magazine's equivocation between science as in-the-making and science as ready-made, *Newsweek* counterbalances public valorization of science with equally intense skepticism and mistrust. The model of science that the magazine advances thus aims to meet conflicting audience demands at the same time: that science be objective and constant, able to access concrete truths about nature, but also be dynamic and responsive to human interests, operating not on high from "Mount Science" (Gieryn, *Cultural Boundaries* 6), but within and in service to the culture that supports it.

Both faces of the science of CAM are persuasive in the public negotiation of biomedical boundaries because each addresses different sets of beliefs about how science works or ought to work. I track these seemingly contradictory perspectives through a rhetorical construction that recurs both implicitly and explicitly across the scholarly and popular literature on biomedical research on CAM. This construction asks, of any given CAM practice, "Does it really work?" This is the implicit central question of randomized controlled trials of CAM, for instance, wherein researchers design studies that can differentiate between interventions that are genuinely effective and those that only just appear to be so via placebo or nonspecific effects. For instance, Bove and Nilsson's trial of chiropractic in *JAMA* discussed in the previous chapter isolated spinal adjustment as the "effective ingredient" in chiropractic treatments, separating it from other elements of chiropractic care to find out if adjustment actually does work.

In popular reporting on complementary and alternative medicine, that key question, "Does it really work?" becomes explicit, often serving as a narrative hook in news stories about the latest trends in health care. *Newsweek*, for one, has long employed this construct: in a 1992 article announcing the launch of the NIH Office of Alternative Medicine, for instance, the magazine asked, "Do remedies like acupuncture and herbal medicine really work?" (Glick 58); five years later, in a 1997 article about zinc for colds, it again asked, "Does it really work?" (Hamilton 48); while in 1999, in an article published in the summer following the *JAMA-Archives* theme issues, the magazine asked, "Can massage, mediation and supplements really improve your health?" ("Weighing Alternatives" 92).

In both scholarly and popular texts that map and blur boundaries between mainstream medicine and CAM, such as the *JAMA-Archives* journals and *Newsweek*, the "Does it really work?" construct is more than a rhetorical question, a question used for effect and not meant to be answered. Rather, this question is what motivates research on CAM and what journalists earnestly seek to answer based on that research. This construct is a useful heuristic for tracing *Newsweek*'s trajectories of persuasion as an instance of biomedical boundary work because it encapsulates the tension between science-in-the-making and ready-made science. A close reading of four such trajectories within the special report will illustrate that, in attempting to answer the question of whether or not CAM really works, *Newsweek* produces a multidimensional model of science that, perhaps counterintuitively, bolsters biomedicine's authority in the public realm and secures its jurisdiction over CAM. These trajectories depict science as (1) an epistemic authority, (2) an independent agent, (3) responsive to social interests, and (4) process-oriented rather than product-oriented. The first two trajectories draw on the view of science as ready-made, while the final two instead draw on a model of science as always, necessarily, in-the-making.

Trajectory One: Science is an epistemic authority. Within the *Newsweek* special report, the most immediate effect of the "Does it really work?" construct is that it positions science as the only legitimate means of separating effective alternative medical interventions from those that are ineffective: Does it *really* work? This trajectory presents science as ready-made, able to adjudicate decisively on age-old folk remedies. In Cowley's lead article, for instance, radiologist Zang-Hee Cho expresses his excitement about the potential of medical scanning technologies to explain acupuncture's effects: "We used to think these were mysterious energies . . . but not anymore. *As we learn how acupuncture really works*, we may find that one well-placed needle can do what we now do with 20" (Cowley 50; emphasis added in this quotation and in those following). The implication here is that science will eventually reveal truths that have eluded us thus far; all we need are the right tests, the right technology. The magazine makes similar claims elsewhere, too. Anne Underwood writes, for example, "If traditional Chinese medicine feels unscientific to the Western mind, that should come as no surprise. Its foundations were laid down more than 2,000 years ago in The Yellow Emperor's Classic of Internal Medicine. *Yet modern science is starting to verify that some of these age-old remedies really work*" ("Learning" 54). Kalb, similarly, reports of new trials of St. John's wort that she says will determine "how safe it *really is*" ("Lift" 68). In these examples, biomedicine's sphere of cultural influence facilitates such claims to epistemic jurisdiction: science has accrued the kind of authority that makes it difficult to imagine a matter, medical or otherwise, about which it could not persuasively adjudicate.

The scientific aim of investigating whether or not CAM interventions work is laudable in itself, but the corollary implication, that only interventions validated by science are meritorious, is one that I demonstrate in chapter 3 is as much the product of concern for professional boundaries as it is for patient safety and care. Considering the vast swaths of everyday biomedical practice that are not evidence-based, it is difficult to defend the idea that CAM practices are suspect simply by virtue of their not having been tested in randomized controlled trials.

Further, the question itself, "Does it really work?" encodes a skepticism not found in its more earnest, unmodified cousin: "Does it work?" In asking whether an intervention *really* works, rather than just seems to, this construct puts CAM users in a tricky spot: those who find benefit from interventions that have not (yet) been validated may, by implication, be imagining things. At the same time, by positioning science as able to assess with final authority effects that patients already experience as real, the construct endows science with an epistemic authority that patients do not themselves possess.

Trajectory Two: Science is an independent agent. As an entity able to penetrate CAM interventions and assess their merits, science also takes on an agency of its own under the "Does it really work?" construct. For example, Underwood explains that "modern science is starting to verify" traditional Chinese medical practices such as herbal remedies and *qigong,* as though science itself were capable of isolating research questions, formulating hypotheses, testing them, and then deriving conclusions based on the data as they are transformed into evidence ("Learning" 54). Similarly, in the deck of Cowley's lead article, the short summary between headline and byline, science plays both investigator and judge: "As science rigorously examines herbs and acupuncture . . ." (47). Such phrasings, which position science as an independent epistemic agent, carry significant rhetorical force, as Randy Allen Harris forcefully notes: "Science has undergone an almost-literal apotheosis, taking over so many of the functions of religion that the primary meaning of *layperson* has shifted from 'non-cleric' to 'non-scientist'. . . . It brings such commanding authority to assertions that we regularly get headlines like 'Science proves Shroud of Turin fake' and 'Science close to cure for AIDS' " (Introduction, *Landmark Essays* xi).

According science an agency of its own powerfully shapes boundary debates, such as that between biomedicine and CAM, because it reinforces the idea that science can answer any question put to it. The first two trajectories of the "Does it really work?" construct in *Newsweek* therefore draw on a model of science as ready-made, under which the question of whether or not CAM practices are safe and effective is straightforward to answer. In this view, although researchers may be fallible, saddled with their own self-interest, science itself appears always on the side of truth. And, as I suggest next with the remaining two trajectories, this is perhaps one of the greatest strengths of the model of science that *Newsweek* evokes in its coverage of CAM research: even when researchers are in a position of weakness, the authority of science itself remains intact.

Trajectory Three: Science is responsive to social interests. As I have argued in previous chapters, the widespread movement over the past two decades of patients beyond biomedicine's boundaries toward CAM has reconfigured the landscape of American health care. This movement has put the medical profession in a somewhat defensive position as it renegotiates its position at the center of that terrain. Although the public was not abandoning mainstream medicine as much as it was embracing CAM simultaneously, mainstream medicine could not help but look culpable as patients flooded natural health stores and alternative medical offices in search of care. Even now, as medicalization reaches further into our lives as ordinary problems of living such as aging are redefined as medical ones (see Conrad), the draw of CAM pulls ever stronger. Reflecting this defensive position, the third trajectory of the "Does it really work?" construct in *Newsweek* is that it situates biomedicine as earnestly asking of CAM: "Does it really *work*?"

The special report depicts scientists as having fallen behind, hurrying to catch up to public interest in CAM. Cowley's article leads by noting, for example, that "after dismissing CAM therapies as quackery for the better part of a century, the medical establishment now finds itself *racing* to evaluate them" (48; emphasis added). Kaptchuk, Eisenberg, and Komaroff similarly explain that "Experts are now *racing* to develop new study designs" to test interventions that are difficult to standardize or control (73; emphasis added). This pattern of scientists racing to catch up recurs elsewhere throughout the special report. One effect of this pattern is that it reduces the authority of science by placing CAM in the lead. However, for individuals who view science and medicine with skepticism, this diminished authority might ultimately reflect positively on science: the image of scientists "racing" to evaluate CAM implies that science reflects and serves the interests of the public. The public leads, and science follows.

Researchers in the *JAMA* and *Archives* theme issues vigorously resisted such a public-oriented model of science, but, in *Newsweek*, the positioning of a weakened medical profession as having falling behind the CAM-consuming public may turn out to be a strength if LaFollette is right that popular magazines can tell us something of what readers believe, or want to believe, about science. Read in this way, *Newsweek* suggests that readers want to believe in a science that is receptive to the public's needs and interests. Trying to catch up to their patients, biomedical practitioners appear, finally, to be listening. Given that many individuals struggle to feel heard within biomedicine, this portrayal of medical researchers as responsive to public demand may secure audience goodwill by presenting a vision of science that appeals to readers' own experiences as patients.[10] To rephrase medical philosopher Miriam Solomon (407), one of the highest praises one can give a physician is to say, "he really *listens* to me."

Certainly, enormous numbers of Americans were already seeking CAM regardless of whether or not the interventions had been rigorously studied, and so the magazine's emphasis on how quickly scientists are racing to study CAM may seem misplaced. Yet, if we keep in mind the first trajectory of the "Does it really work?" construct, that science has a special acuity of vision that allows it to see what members of the public cannot, then researchers' efforts to evaluate CAM through scientific principles are reframed as a response to public demand, even if the public does not know well enough to make that demand.

In the service of this framing of science as responsive to public interest, a high level of activity runs through *Newsweek*'s special report. The state of research on CAM is described in terms of movement and abundance as scientists mobilize a swift response to a public exigence. With the founding of NCCAM, for instance, Cowley reports that "the money and excitement *spread quickly*" (48), resulting in a "*flurry* of research" (53; emphasis added). Many of the articles describe studies in rapid-fire succession, placing the reader in the middle of the action in a bustling field of research. Kalb, for example, describes sixteen different clinical trials in her 1,500-word article, which consequently reads like a list of abstracts ("Lift"). Similarly, Mary Carmichael situates the abundant studies that she reports on as occurring simultaneously: "A six-year trial started in 1999 will likely yield more definite answers. *Meanwhile*, doctors are also studying the compounds often mixed with ginkgo . . ."

(57; emphasis added). Although these articles frequently caution that more studies are needed before we can draw firm conclusions whether or not a given intervention works (see Kalb, "Lift" 70 and "Natural" 65; Noonan 60), there seems in *Newsweek* to be an embarrassment of riches in biomedical research on CAM. Although scientists are breathlessly playing catch-up, science itself appears to have everything under control: studies are underway, the magazine assures us, and the resulting evidence will be available soon.

Trajectory Four: Science is process-oriented, not product-oriented. The question of evidence complicates the picture of science in *Newsweek* because, even though the field of CAM research is bustling, there never seems to be enough evidence to confirm whether or not a given intervention really does work. Accordingly, as an epistemic agent, science is able to give us reliable knowledge about the natural world, but that knowledge is always necessarily provisional, subject to revision—it is only reliable *for now*. Study data are frequently reported in the magazine under heavy qualification, just as they would be in scientific journals: "Several *small* studies have found . . ."; "exercise *may* ease . . . symptoms"; "*preliminary* evidence *suggests*" (Weiger and Eisenberg 49; emphasis added). Even when there is established evidence for a given intervention, there is always room for more. Carmichael notes, for example, that although "ginkgo is one of the most thoroughly examined remedies in complementary medicine, the verdict isn't in yet" (57), while Shmerling and colleagues describe data on CAM for osteoarthritis as still too limited: "rigorous evidence is still lacking"; "scientific evidence is too sparse"; and "its benefits are not well established" (53). Even when there seems to be an abundance of studies on a given intervention, as in Kalb's report on a meta-analysis of twenty-nine clinical trials of natural hot-flash treatments, there remain only "small amounts of reliable data so far" despite the seemingly large number of trials that have been conducted ("Natural" 65).

In these articles about CAM research, science is process-oriented: knowledge in-the-making unfolds over time rather than arriving ready-made, free of problems or context. In one view, the inherent instability of that knowledge as it is revised and refined through standard scientific processes may undermine the available evidence on CAM. A skeptic could say, "Well, what do scientists know anyway? Whatever they say today, they'll contradict with a new study tomorrow." But an alternate reading, consistent with the magazine's overall position that science will ultimately succeed in determining which CAM interventions work, is that the uncertainty of scientific knowledge in *Newsweek* places a premium on evidence that is able to withstand those processes. Like extracting gold from ore, such processes consume a lot of time, energy, and expense, and their output ("data") is considerably smaller than their waste (i.e., the many trials whose results are insufficient, inconclusive, or invalid). In this framework, the prospect of producing reliable data is rendered extremely valuable by virtue of its rarity and expense.

In asking of CAM, "Does it really work?" the *Newsweek* special report ultimately bolsters science's epistemic authority, but not along lines predictable from the rhetorical scholarship on popular science. While popular reporting about science generally demonstrates high levels of certainty, avoiding qualifiers and emphasizing research products rather than processes, *Newsweek* instead tends toward uncertainty. By qualifying research evidence and questioning the limits of its application, the magazine exposes what Angela Cassidy calls the "messy internal face of science" (175), where knowledge on a given issue remains unsettled and debates about scientific practice spill over into the public realm.

If we consider the *Newsweek* special report as an episode of biomedical boundary work, then the unsettling of scientific knowledge within its pages may have distinct effects among (at least) two populations of the magazine's readers. For scientists and physicians, particularly those concerned about the potential impact of the research on their profession or practice, the high levels of uncertainty expressed in the magazine would align with their own professional values and characteristic styles of expression. For popular readers who are skeptical of science and its ability to adjudicate fairly on the effectiveness of CAM, the high levels of uncertainty in the magazine may signify a humbler, wiser science, one that is less territorial and more open to inquiry. For both sets of readers, *Newsweek* could be seen as making a case for the legitimacy of scientific research on CAM.[11] Although the special report does diminish the authority of science as scientists "race" to catch up to CAM, that authority nevertheless enables science—and only science—to determine whether or not a given CAM intervention really works. Following on Bradley Lewis's analysis of *Newsweek*'s 2001 biotechnology issue, I would argue likewise that, in its coverage of CAM research, the magazine "encode[s] a somewhat ambivalent but still highly medicalized reading position" (373).

In this section, I have described what I identify as the four main persuasive trajectories of the "Does it really work?" construct in public discourse about CAM: that it positions science as the only legitimate instrument for evaluating whether CAM interventions actually do work, that it gives science an agency of its own to weigh in on epistemic matters, that it facilitates the magazine's depiction of science as attendant to the public's interests, and that it underscores the necessarily tentative nature of scientific evidence and the need for ever more research. While the first two of these trajectories call upon a model of science as ready-made, the remaining two call upon a more complex understanding of scientific processes and practices.

I have used these trajectories as heuristics, to sketch out the model of science that underlies the *Newsweek* special report, which turns out to be quite different from the integrative model of the "new science" of CAM about which the magazine ostensibly reports. In the context of professional boundary work in popular media, one of the most significant implications of this model of science, which draws on both of the two faces of science, is that, by incorporating seemingly oppositional characteristics of science into a single, coherent model, the *Newsweek* report makes it hard to imagine that anything but science could determine, unequivocally, whether or not CAM "really works."

Mapping Boundaries of Expertise in *Newsweek*

The first two sections of this chapter examined the broader contours of the *Newsweek* special report, approaching medical reporting as a variety of science reporting. In those sections, I did not differentiate among the report's authors, who hold varying levels of scientific expertise. The remaining two sections sharpen my focus on boundary work within the magazine by examining popular medicine as an exceptional, rather than a typical, case in popular science. I develop that claim by showing how popular science *by* scientists might usefully be considered separately from that by journalists and other authors.

In this chapter's introduction, I discussed some of the crucial differences between popular science and popular medicine. These differences rest largely on the particular kinds of expertise the public brings to popular texts on health and medicine, and on how the ideas that are circulated in those texts manage also to circulate beyond individual readers. An additional distinction I want to make is among different kinds of authors, a distinction that is often overlooked in studies of popularization. Questions about speakers—about their character, their position in relation to both their texts and audiences, and the contexts within which they speak—have always been central in rhetorical study but, while analyses of popular science have paid good attention to the matter of who is being addressed in popular science, questions about the speakers themselves have often been flattened out. The *Newsweek* special report is a good place to illustrate these differences among speakers with different rhetorical investments because the articles were produced under largely "controlled" circumstances: they were published in the same venue, on the same rhetorical occasion, under the same (or similar) editorial conditions, and for the same audience, but they were written by different sorts of authors. While the articles do vary by genre and by subject, their identical context and audience can isolate how categories of authorship factor into popular accounts of biomedical research.

I take my cue in these final two sections from questions that Judy Segal asks of breast cancer narratives: "what do breast cancer stories *do* when they circulate in public life? What do they do *for* us and what do they do *to* us?" ("Breast Cancer" 6; original emphasis). One of the things such stories do, Segal argues, is produce and maintain ignorance about breast cancer by making some stories more tellable than others. The stories that we cannot tell, the stories that are suppressed, she argues, narrate breast cancer differently; examining what those untellable stories say and how they are suppressed can highlight the radical limits of public discourse about breast cancer. Segal's examination of this discourse demonstrates how we—as bodies, as people— can be invisibly restoried in public discourse and then have those stories returned to us as *our* stories.[12] The story of biomedical CAM research that is told in the *Newsweek* special report similarly overwrites other stories that could have been told, stories that seem better to match the concerns and interests of the magazine's target audience, the majority of which consumes or has consumed complementary and alternative medicine. One factor underlying the suppression of certain elements of the story of CAM research, I suggest, has significantly to do with the nature of medical reporting itself, particularly the conflicting demands its writers face such as the need to accommodate their readers' expert knowledge about some aspects of health and medicine but lack of expertise about others.

In this section, I examine the role of expertise in the *Newsweek* special report. The once-prevalent view of popular science held that audiences are separated by a vast deficit or gap from the expert knowledge of scientists and that the work of science journalism was to translate that knowledge for consumption by an "ignorant and dependent" public (Bensaude-Vincent 101). Scholars in rhetoric and science studies have since discounted this unidirectional "deficit model," arguing that the contexts and effects of popular science are far more varied, and the public more informed and invested as an audience, than the deficit model allows.[13] I argue here that this is particularly true of popular medicine, that audiences of popular reporting on health, illness, and treatment have a specific kind of expertise simply by virtue of being audiences at all. While not everyone will have knowledge about recent advances in mechanical engineering or particle physics, all are expert on the experience of being a person with a body, one that is sometimes sick, sometimes in pain. This form of embodied expertise shifts the rhetorical dynamic of popular medicine, adding weight to the place of audience in the classic rhetorical triangle of speaker-text-audience. While all three elements of this triangle exist in tension in all rhetorical contexts, the balance in popular medicine tips toward the audience to a greater extent than it does in popular science.

The distinction I am making between popular science and popular medicine is not simply that expertise is more important in the latter context than in the former because readers have more knowledge of health and medicine than they do of physics or biotechnology or engineering. Rather, my greater concern is that, as Peter Broks reminds us, "we cannot extricate popular science . . . from wider issues of power, authority and the demarcation of what is science from what is not" (123). Popular medicine is embedded in that same matrix of "power, authority, and . . . demarcation," but its stakes are higher because readers' own embodied forms of expertise are suspended within and defined by that matrix. Even a person who does not follow popular stories about health and medicine can be affected by those stories as they circulate and become dominant cultural narratives about illness and health that answer the question "How shall I be ill?" (Segal, "Sexualization" 369). The *Newsweek* special report is a fruitful site for examining these forms of expertise in popular medicine because it re-presents CAM practices, in biomedical terms, to the public that precipitated the research on CAM. Mapping how these popular texts negotiate expertise can help us further track boundary work in medicine because it shows that, despite the prevalence of rhetorics of empowerment in public discourse on health and medicine, some forms of expertise are more valuable in popular texts than are others.

The idea that there is a gap between scientists and the rest of society permeates the *Newsweek* special report, whether or not that idea is valid. The very arrangement of the report promotes this view, with the "Insights from Harvard Medical School" sections differentiated visually from the rest of the articles (see fig. 7). Set within clearly delineated text boxes against a contrastive yellow background, each "Insight" features artwork depicting the region of the body discussed in the text (upper body, leg, torso), with x-ray style geometric shapes superimposed that reveal the underlying location of pathology (cells in the body, bones of the knee, vertebrae). This artwork literalizes the metaphor that doctors can "see" inside our bodies: through imaging technologies, they can know our bodies in ways that we cannot. These specialized ways of knowing about patients' bodies effectively shut patients out of their own care, with diagnoses often made via x-rays and scans in the patient's absence.[14] One of the byproducts of medicine's specialized gaze, as Foucault notes, is that the very act of being seen changes us. In this case, the artwork serves as a

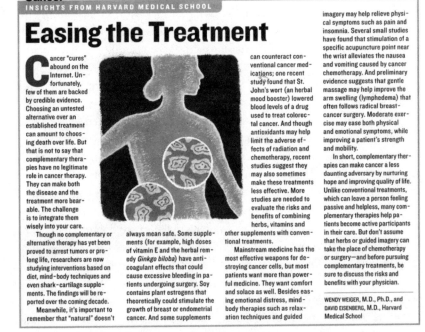

Cancer
INSIGHTS FROM HARVARD MEDICAL SCHOOL

Easing the Treatment

Cancer "cures" abound on the Internet. Unfortunately, few of them are backed by credible evidence. Choosing an untested alternative over an established treatment can amount to choosing death over life. But that is not to say that complementary therapies have no legitimate role in cancer therapy. They can make both the disease and the treatment more bearable. The challenge is to integrate them wisely into your care.

Though no complementary or alternative therapy has yet been proved to arrest tumors or prolong life, researchers are now studying interventions based on diet, mind-body techniques and even shark-cartilage supplements. The findings will be reported over the coming decade.

Meanwhile, it's important to remember that "natural" doesn't always mean safe. Some supplements (for example, high doses of vitamin E and the herbal remedy *Ginkgo biloba*) have anticoagulant effects that could cause excessive bleeding in patients undergoing surgery. Soy contains plant estrogens that theoretically could stimulate the growth of breast or endometrial cancer. And some supplements can counteract conventional cancer medications; one recent study found that St. John's wort (an herbal mood booster) lowered blood levels of a drug used to treat colorectal cancer. And though antioxidants may help limit the adverse effects of radiation and chemotherapy, recent studies suggest they may also sometimes make these treatments less effective. More studies are needed to evaluate the risks and benefits of combining herbs, vitamins and other supplements with conventional treatments.

Mainstream medicine has the most effective weapons for destroying cancer cells, but most patients want more than powerful medicine. They want comfort and solace as well. Besides easing emotional distress, mind-body therapies such as relaxation techniques and guided imagery may help relieve physical symptoms such as pain and insomnia. Several small studies have found that stimulation of a specific acupuncture point near the wrist alleviates the nausea and vomiting caused by cancer chemotherapy. And preliminary evidence suggests that gentle massage may help improve the arm swelling (lymphedema) that often follows radical breast-cancer surgery. Moderate exercise may ease both physical and emotional symptoms, while improving a patient's strength and mobility.

In short, complementary therapies can make cancer a less daunting adversary by nurturing hope and improving quality of life. Unlike conventional treatments, which can leave a person feeling passive and helpless, many complementary therapies help patients become active participants in their care. But don't assume that herbs or guided imagery can take the place of chemotherapy or surgery—and before pursuing complementary treatments, be sure to discuss the risks and benefits with your physician.

WENDY WEIGER, M.D., Ph.D., and
DAVID EISENBERG, M.D., Harvard
Medical School

FIGURE 7. "Cancer: Insights from Harvard Medical School," James Steinberg, *Newsweek* 2 Dec. 2002: 49.

reminder that medical specialists can see us better than we can see ourselves. For *Newsweek* readers who use and value CAM, the stark differentiation between their ability to know their own bodies and medical practitioners' ability to know those same bodies brings into focus the transformation that CAM undergoes in its encounter with science.

The gap in the *Newsweek* report between experts and nonexperts is also maintained by the use of credentials, which further differentiate the articles by researchers from those by journalists. All but one of the "Insights from Harvard Medical School" text boxes list their authors' doctoral-level degrees and professional affiliations, while the longer feature article by medical researchers Kaptchuk, Eisenberg, and Komaroff ("Pondering") lists the authors' association with Harvard Medical School. The one exception in the Harvard "Insights" is the article on the placebo effect that is coauthored by Ted Kaptchuk, whose professional designation is OMD (Doctor of Oriental Medicine). He and coauthors Eisenberg and Komaroff, both MDs, are listed not by degree but by title: "*Drs.* Ted Kaptchuk, David Eisenberg, and Anthony Komaroff, Harvard Medical School" (73; emphasis added). Given how similar the Harvard "Insights" are otherwise (layout, style, graphics, tone, content, and purpose), and given the parallel construction in the listing of all the other expert authors (name, degree, affiliation), this exception stands out. Its intent may have been to emphasize Kaptchuk's status as *doctor* rather than as *TCM Practitioner*.[15] Even still, what is key in these examples is that none of the journalist-authored articles list the authors' qualifications, while all of the researcher-authored articles do. The implication is that the expert-authors are authorities we can trust.

The special report also draws lines of distinction between experts and nonexperts through pronouns such as "us," "them," "we," and "they," aligning the magazine's journalist-authors with the public and differentiating all of us, as a collective, from the expert-authors. The journalist-authors use inclusive pronouns to establish common ground with their readers, a convention of popular science (Dowdey): "In this Special Report, NEWSWEEK explores how acupuncture, herbs, tai chi and biofeedback have many doctors reexamining how *they* treat all of *us*" ("Top of the Week" 3; emphasis added). Notably, "treat" takes on a double connotation here, as in *Please treat my headache, doctor* but also as in *Please don't treat me like that*. This double meaning explains the high levels of public interest in CAM as largely the result of patient dissatisfaction with biomedicine, an explanation that is reinforced in many of the articles.

Journalist Cowley also identifies himself inclusively as one of us: "*We* make more visits to nonconventional healers . . . than *we* do to MDs," he says, "and *we* spend more of *our* own money for the privilege" (48, emphasis added). Our distance from those holding the keys to biomedicine becomes clearer later in that same paragraph, as we are told that "*the* medical establishment now finds *itself* racing to evaluate . . ." (48). Researcher-authored articles also reinforce this distance between scientists and the public by addressing readers in the second person, in exclusive terms of "you" rather than "us." The "Harvard Insights," for example, advise readers to "integrate [CAM] wisely into *your* care" (Weiger and Eisenberg 49), warning that taking herbal remedies for depression "may serve *you* well. *But be careful*" (Craig Miller; first emphasis added, second in original). While the journalist-authors generally speak as one of us, that is, the researcher-authors generally speak *to* us.

In the researcher-authored articles, the experts behave exactly as we might expect: they speak with ease as physicians talking to patients. They write in a manner that might best be described through Bourdieu's assertion that there exists in linguistic production a certain "*relaxation in tension*" in which speakers "endow their linguistic performances with a casualness and ease that are precisely recognized as the hallmark of distinction in such matters," thereby asserting their authority within the speech situation (659;

original emphasis). None of the researcher-authors in *Newsweek* refer to any specific studies or researchers, aside from the well-known Harvard Nurses' Health Study (in Haskell and Eisenberg), whereas the journalists overwhelmingly do provide such identifying information, including researchers' names and institutional affiliations. Language researchers de Oliveira and Pagano note that lack of citation, direct or indirect, is an indication that an author of popular science feels "comfortable enough" with the material that he or she sees no need to bolster claims by pointing to an authorizing source (642). The pace of the expert-articles is also measurably slower, less frantic, than the journalist-authored pieces. Collectively, the expert-authors each assume the tone of an experienced doctor explicitly offering advice to a patient, usually in the form of lists that keep the lines of transmission clear, from doctor to advice-seeking patient: "Here are some potential remedies . . ." (Shmerling, Ulbricht, and Basch).

The researcher-authored articles also express a firm conviction that *Newsweek*'s readers find biomedical examination of CAM not only desirable but also necessary. The special report is shot through with a vision of CAM as an undiscovered country or frontier that the ambassadors of scientific medicine are hard at work mapping and analyzing, as if to clear the territory for public travel. The "live-on-location" feel of the report's account of the intense research activity surrounding CAM contributes to this impression to the extent that it is not hard to imagine scientists racing by with theodolites and GPS receivers as they rush to map the terrain.

For the Harvard "Insights," for example, the key assumption seems to be that readers, now framed as patients, will go out into the newly mapped world of CAM and use these text boxes as guides for navigating the territory. Shmerling, Ulbricht, and Basch's list of arthritis remedies reads like a travel guidebook, for example, briefly describing the state of research on five remedies and pointing out which ones are worth stopping at and checking out, and which we should just drive past. Frontier metaphors, common in emerging areas of science (Ceccarelli, *Frontier*, "Mixed Metaphors"; Nelkin), appeal to high civic ideals such as adventure and the expansion of knowledge, but frontiers can also be dangerous places, especially for those who previously occupied the territory. If we consider the specific, embodied expertise that audiences bring to popular medicine, we might find that these new scientific maps of CAM overdetermine the terrain they attempt to represent. We might also find that these maps may not, in fact, be wanted at all.

I argued in the introduction to this chapter that one of the *Newsweek* special report's most notable features is that it returned the products of CAM research to the same public that motivated it. As previous chapters have shown,

CAM is transformed as it is mapped with biomedical tools, and those seeking CAM may not find in this new biomedically approved version the same qualities that brought them to CAM in the first place. As Ceccarelli observes, regarding map metaphors in genetics, "A map that surveys the frontier is designed to open up a territory for settlement and for development, to make it possible for its owners to conquer the land for use and for profit. Although it represents things the way they are now, it does so with the express purpose of aiding in the alteration of that territory" ("Mixed Metaphors" 98–99). One of the stories that does not get told in the *Newsweek* report is the story of what happens to CAM as it is mapped by biomedicine, as it is settled and (re)developed, and, in turn, what happens to the individuals who valued the freedom to navigate the terrain on their own. The gulf between expert and nonexpert widens as these individuals are told in the magazine simply, "Talk to your doctor."

Displaced Stories about CAM and CAM Research

As a means of exploring some of the other stories not told in the *Newsweek* special report about biomedical research on CAM, I now turn to the journalist-authored articles. The authors of these articles are positioned at the intersection of various interests, including those of expert informants, administrative and regulatory bodies, advertisers, editors, and readers, as well as entrenched public values about the place and purpose of science within North American culture. Collectively, these journalist-authored articles consist of two intertwined narratives: a narrative of research activity and a narrative of the people that use CAM. These two narratives correspond, respectively, with two key features of popular science identified by theorists such as Fahnestock, Nelkin, and Bruce Lewenstein: that science journalists internalize scientific values (an expectation met by the narrative of research activity) and that they appeal, explicitly, to the interests and values of their readers (met by the narrative of CAM users). As I have noted above, Segal argues that narrative itself serves a regulatory function in public discourse about breast cancer, in which the emergence of a "standard story" makes other stories harder to tell ("Breast Cancer"). In this section, I examine the *Newsweek* report's two interwoven narratives of research activity and the people who use CAM as standard stories that effectively suppress other possible narratives of surrounding CAM. These standard stories point to larger tensions underlying the negotiation of medical-professional boundaries in popular medicine.

The first narrative in the *Newsweek* report, about research activity, is less about individual trials of CAM than it is about research itself. This narrative makes a claim about what sort of enterprise science is, particularly in its emphasis on bustling activity in the research field. As I suggested earlier, this story of research does not conform to arguments in scholarship on popular science that science journalists suppress areas of dissent and present knowledge as ready-made. Scientific knowledge is portrayed in *Newsweek* as necessarily tentative, and I think we can read this portrayal of science as in-the-making as evidence that scientific values are strongly internalized within the articles. That is, when talking about the biomedical knowledge base on CAM, the journalists in *Newsweek* often sound like scientists themselves, qualifying what we do know and carefully explaining what we do not know. The journalists are notably cautious about generalizing findings, emphasizing the often provisional nature of scientific evidence.[16] These emphases on scientific values may be strategic: by sounding like scientists, the authors may seek to enhance their ethos, and by appearing faithful to the ideals of science, they may seek to nurture working relationships with their scientific informants.

In the other set of narratives in the *Newsweek* special report, we hear stories—many stories—about people that use CAM and have uniformly benefited from it. We hear about Sheldon and Tosha Janz (Noonan), for example, who responded to their pediatrician's suggestion that their two-year-old take steroids for asthma by seeking a second opinion; the second physician agreed with the first. Undaunted, they sought a third opinion, this time from a doctor of integrative medicine, who suggested that they cut dairy products from their son's diet and, upon following that suggestion, the toddler's wheezing promptly stopped. We hear about Marisa Harris, fifty-four, who had refused chemotherapy and was given nine months to live but then joined a meditation class and support group, which changed her mind about chemotherapy. Now, Cowley reports, "Four years later, she's as happy as she has ever been in her life" (52). We hear about Ann Moffat, fifty, the woman from the hot dog stand who felt she had received such a strong benefit in a clinical trial of black cohosh for hot flashes that she began taking it once the trial was over, even though she admits to not knowing whether she received a placebo or the real thing (Kalb, "Natural"); we hear about Christie Blackwood, the preteen whose chemotherapy-related nausea was controlled by guided imagery; and we hear about many others besides.

All of these stories in the *Newsweek* special report, together, are remarkable in several ways. First, their volume alone is dizzying: we hear about a lot of people that use CAM. But, second, we do not learn a lot about any of them, as the stories are told in the same rapid-fire style in which the research stories are told. We hear about this patient and that one, but we end up knowing nothing much about any of them. If we wanted to transcribe a general formula for each of these stories, it might go something like this: *[Name], [age], could not find relief for [condition] so s/he tried [CAM practice] and now feels better (than ever)*. What are the functions of these stories? Individually, they offer points of identification for readers, perhaps allowing them to recognize themselves within the larger story about the new science of CAM. The personal stories also humanize the research narrative, providing contrast to its institutional flavor. These stories appeal to popular interests and values by, for example, portraying CAM, which so many Americans use, in a positive light. The personal stories also contribute to the authors' ethos by conveying the sense that, despite all the journalist-authors' talk about placebos and multi-armed trials and the generalizability of results, they really are "one of us." Note, for instance, that none of the researcher-authored articles feature personal stories.

Together, these individual personal stories add up to a larger narrative, one that essentially says that CAM seekers are regular people motivated by good reasons and have received both help and solace from the CAM practices they have sought. This larger narrative bolsters the special report's announcement of the arrival of the new, integrative medicine. However, this narrative seems also to be an effort to placate CAM-using readers that may be disappointed to find out how few CAM interventions have been proven safe and effective, as well as to keep advertisers happy, since the report is peppered with advertisements for dietary supplements such as megavitamins, black cohosh, and soy isoflavones. Both of these strategies point to larger tensions underlying rhetorics of popular science and medicine.

The two narratives in the *Newsweek* special report, about CAM research and CAM users, offer what Segal might call "standard stories" about the science of alternative medicine. These dominant narratives suppress other narratives that might be told, narratives that reveal a more complex view of the culture of health and medicine. What these stories *do not* tell us about medicine can sometimes reveal far more than what they *do* tell. Working within the framework that Segal and others, such as Broks and Carolyn Michelle, have outlined, I want to highlight, in closing, some of those suppressed stories and suggest what they might mean regarding how the notion of evidence is mobilized in arguments about the boundaries of biomedicine.

With respect to the narrative of medical research, we learn that scientists race, that scientific work takes perseverance through trial and error, and that scientific evidence is valuable for being difficult to obtain and expensive to produce. However, we do not hear about why scientists are "racing" in the first place—or rather, we do not hear the whole story about it, the one that embeds very legitimate concerns about patient safety and health within the larger web of motivations governing biomedical research on CAM. One such concern, for example, is protecting professional jurisdiction, an issue I examined in chapter 2. We also do not learn in *Newsweek* about the limits of and barriers to research on CAM. Constructing science as an almost omniscient power offers readers the sense that, given enough time and money, science can get to the bottom of anything. If we do not have answers on a particular question, the *Newsweek* special report suggests, it only means that we do not have them *yet*. Although some articles do describe methodological barriers in CAM research, such as the problems of randomization and placebo controls (Kaptchuk, Eisenberg, and Komaroff, "Pondering"), none engage with the professional disincentives that researchers on CAM might face in their research. Such problems include securing funding for their studies (especially given that so much funding now comes from pharmaceutical companies), finding appropriate scholarly venues in which to publish their research (since CAM studies are still often perceived as suspect or poorly designed), and maintaining their own professional credibility as scientists studying interventions and practices that have uncertain status in biomedicine.

The articles similarly deflect the role of politics in research, a strategy that Nelkin identifies as common practice in popular science. Noonan, for instance, criticizes the FDA for its "lack of regulation" of dietary supplements such as herbal remedies and high-dose vitamins but fails to point out that, under the Dietary Supplement Health and Education Act (DSHEA), the FDA actually does not have jurisdiction over them. DSHEA was legislated in response to public demand and heavy lobbying from the supplement industry, in the face of vigorous opposition by the American Medical Association (as detailed in chapter 4). Glossing over this history, Noonan instead describes biomedical researchers in heroic terms, as willing to step in and do the FDA's work in order to save the public from being "lured with false promises and bogus claims" (62). Although the *Newsweek* report features only individuals that have benefited from CAM, there is a shadowy sense across the articles that consumers must be wary and protect themselves by choosing only practices that have been cleared for use by biomedical researchers.

The many individual stories we hear about patients in the magazine perform similar deflecting functions. Segal observes that the dominant breast cancer narrative, as a genre with conventionalized features, stifles stories of women with breast cancer who are not energetic optimists, those who do not become better people as a result of their disease, and those who die. In the *Newsweek* special report, we see a similar pattern. There are no stories, for example,

of those who feel they have been defrauded or those who were injured or became sick as a result of their CAM use. We do not hear from people who resent
being told to ask their doctors about health interventions they have used for
years without physician approval. We hear a lot about risk, about whether or
not CAM practices are safe, but, as Broks points out, the danger of risk-talk is
that we end up "asking simply whether a technology is safe rather than whether
it is necessary" (126).

Broks' question anticipates perhaps the biggest question that is obscured
by the personal stories in the *Newsweek* theme issue: Why is all of this medicine, alternative or not, necessary in the first place?

This question is essentially "crowded out," to use Carolyn Michelle's
phrase (62), by a stream of happy CAM users, such as the women in the Kalb
article on menopause treatments whose photographs I discussed earlier in
this chapter. Michelle investigates "anecdotal personalization" in media discourse on cord-blood banking programs, which prominently feature testimo-
nials from parents who express both their relief that they have secured their
child's future health and their gratitude to CordBank for making that future
possible. Michelle's observation that "anecdotal personalization privileges the
experiences and testimony of individuals at the expense of in-depth interro-
gation and critique" (62) resonates with Segal's concern that stories praising
individual health habits (such as those of Sheryl Crow, who "never skips her
vitamins" [7]) and individual health triumphs via rhetorics of "survivorship"
silence other important stories, such as stories about environmental carcino-
gens (see also Kopelson; Pezzullo).

Part of the emphasis on individually oriented explanations of illness, as
both Michelle and Segal point out, links back to neoliberal consumer values
and to the idea that we are solely responsible, for better or worse, for our own
health (Derkatch, "Wellness"; Henwood, Harris, and Spoel). In the case of
Newsweek, we do not hear, for instance, about the cultural conditions that
make it possible to think of menopause as a medical condition requiring
treatment. With the evidence suggesting that hormone replacement therapy
may do more harm than good, women are depicted in Kalb's article as essentially stranded, desperately in need of treatment, as though menopause were
a condition from which one could die. I do not wish to diminish the very real
discomfort that women experience during menopause, but the suppression
of these kinds of questions about CAM, about what it ultimately means to
bring CAM under the purview of biomedicine, has consequences that play
out in the bodies of CAM users themselves.

I would argue further that the increased movement toward complemen-

tary and alternative medicine over the past several decades, and the consequent impulse to test CAM interventions scientifically, speaks to just how
invested we are in scientific frames of thinking. Widespread public interest in
CAM practitioners and therapies is good evidence that we have so embraced
the idea that health can and ought to be restored and maintained via external
intervention that when mainstream medicine does not provide the relief we
seek, we search for other cures when we might do better, at least sometimes,
to reframe our understanding of the issues that affect us.

One could argue, for example, that rather than simply trying to fight bodily
states such as menopause, chronic pain, sleep problems, and stress through
new and better pills (pharmaceutical or herb) and practitioners (mainstream
or alternative), we might rethink our approach, individually and collectively,
to how we interpret and respond to these bodily states. We might also attend
more fully to the ways that we structure and engage in our daily lives within
the reality that we are all, ultimately, bodies in process. The exuberance with
which *Newsweek* reports on the new science of CAM, then, suggests not a
break with bioscientific, pharmaceutically oriented frameworks of health and
illness that emphasize the application of research evidence to the treatment
of bodily failure but, rather, a deeper investment in those same frameworks.

*

Fahnestock's early work on science popularization argued that popular science is primarily epideictic, in the sense that it celebrates and reinscribes
conventional scientific values. This is certainly true in many contexts but, for
biomedical boundary work, I would suggest that, more importantly, popular
science and medicine also map *cultural* values onto those scientific values.
The *Newsweek* special report on scientific research on complementary and
alternative medicine, for instance, praises individualistic qualities such as
pioneerism, savvy, and steely determination, exemplified by the Janz family,
who bucked conventional medical wisdom regarding their son's asthma and
found a doctor who would listen to them.

But the *Newsweek* report couches the exemplars of those individualistic qualities—the patients, practitioners, and researchers depicted in the
magazine—within narratives that simultaneously reinscribe science's hege-
monic influence on North American life, such as a neoliberal emphasis on
consumer behavior and individual health habits. Revealingly, for example,
the Janzes conducted their experiment with CAM under the safety of a doctor's supervision. These narratives stress, ultimately, the necessity of risk-
avoidance and tightly controlled consumer activity and the importance of

public respect for hierarchy and expertise—respect, that is, for science. The "new science" of CAM is not, then, a CAM that has become scientific itself. Rather, it is a CAM that has been absorbed into science.

The borders between biomedicine and CAM that materialize in the *Newsweek* special report mirror those within the *JAMA-Archives* theme issues that I have examined over the course of this book. In both cases, biomedicine emerges from its boundary encounter with CAM reinvigorated, with a wider scope, perhaps, but still recognizable as biomedicine. The model of CAM that is returned in the *Newsweek* report, filtered through science, to the public that it serves illuminates how boundary work operates beyond the limits of upstream science. It shows, for instance, how science and scientists can be challenged by the public's interest in CAM and yet maintain their position of authority.

The remaking of both science and medicine in popular contexts is persuasive because it conditions how we think about how they operate as systems of knowledge and practice and about how they affect our lives. Further, studying the boundaries between biomedicine and CAM as they emerge, differently, within the same "discourse moment" (Moirand) can help us to think in more complex terms about popular science and popular medicine as related but distinct rhetorical phenomena. Biomedical boundary work occurs at all points along the spectrum of science both upstream and downstream. As this chapter has argued, popular reporting on CAM research is a crucial site for the "repeated and endless edging and filling" of biomedical boundaries (Gieryn, *Cultural Boundaries* 14) because popular reports do not only reinforce boundaries drawn further upstream: they also draw boundaries of their own.

Boundaries as Entry Points

In February 2014, as I neared completion of the draft of this book, the Canadian daily newspaper the *Globe and Mail* published a profile of the Brampton Naturopathic Teaching Clinic, the first hospital-based clinic of its kind in Canada, located just outside of Toronto in the province of Ontario. Health reporter Kelly Grant cited the clinic's founding the previous summer as evidence of naturopathy's growing legitimacy in the country's health care system. This shift toward legitimation, Grant reported, would be ratified later in 2014, when Ontario became the second Canadian province (after British Columbia) to allow naturopaths to order a range of laboratory tests and prescribe certain pharmaceuticals. Grant's article provides an even-handed assessment of this legislative development, quoting excited naturopaths and patients alongside concerned medical professionals and organizations, including the Ontario Medical Association, the College of Physicians and Surgeons, and the *Canadian Medical Association Journal*, all of which expressed apprehension about the inclusion of naturopathic approaches to health within a biomedical framework.

The day after the *Globe* story ran, Canada's competing daily newspaper, the *National Post*, fired a shot at Grant's coverage of naturopathy. Columnist Jonathan Kay accused Grant of boostering "pseudoscience" and "celebrat[ing] the legitimization of . . . a bunch of placebo doctors," a move that Kay asserts is nothing short of irresponsible:

The line between science and pseudoscience is a very real and important one. It's the line we depend on, from a public-health perspective, when doctors assure parents that vaccines don't cause autism. It's the line we depend on when doctors tell their patients that, no, those mail-order vitamins they bought on the internet won't negate the effects of smoking. Any move that serves to blur that line is a move that, indirectly at least, endangers public health.

Kay argues that the progressive enfranchisement of complementary and alternative medicine "is a mistake" unsupported by "state-of-the-art, scientific, evidence-based, peer-reviewed medical standards."

Kay's assessment of naturopathy here draws virtually the same line separating science from nonscience, on the same principles, as the one that was drawn by the editors of the *JAMA* and *Archives* coordinated CAM-themed issues some sixteen years earlier.[1] The continued framing of the distinction between biomedicine and CAM as simply one between science and nonscience (or phony science) indicates that much of the discourse surrounding CAM has become locked in a pattern that reduces historically complex and socially contingent processes into a neat binary. Framed in such a pattern, our collective understanding of what counts as a safe, effective health treatment, alternative or not, is constrained by the terms of the debate itself. Only through a comprehensive, textured understanding of these terms will we have the insight necessary to understand how the boundaries of biomedicine are made and remade over time and across contexts. As I have shown in the preceding chapters, what seem at first in biomedical discourse about CAM to be problems of theory, method, and practice are rooted deeply in the rhetorical and generic structures of medicine itself.

Over the course of this book, I have examined scientific research on alternative medicine through rhetorician Kenneth Burke's metaphor of photographic filters, or "terministic screens," to answer this question: *How does the notion of evidence determine the boundaries of biomedicine, from expert to public contexts?* I have viewed the *JAMA* and *Archives* coordinated theme issues on CAM and their related textual artifacts as a collective snapshot that captures the medical profession's boundary-negotiating discursive activity at a particular moment in time. Following my initial chapter, which established my main arguments, each subsequent chapter examined biomedical boundary work through a different filter: the historical-professional, the epistemological, the clinical, and the public. Each filter in turn revealed different aspects of medicine—and of rhetoric.

Chapter 1 established the larger context within which the "rhetorical moment" of the *JAMA-Archives* theme issues on CAM unfolded. I examined the transition from a model of medicine premised on the clinical expertise of individual practitioners to evidence-based medicine, which places research-derived evidence from randomized controlled trials at the center of medical decision-making. I showed how the historical boundaries between mainstream medicine and alternative health practices had been fluid, shaped more by professional negotiation and jurisdiction-seeking than by empirical evidence regarding the validity of one practice or practitioner over another. With the rise of the clinical trial and its ability to determine with unprecedented rigor and precision the safety and efficacy of a given health practice, the boundaries separating biomedicine from health practices that lacked quantifiable evidence of their effects grew ever stronger—and the medical profession, ever more powerful.

The second and third chapters highlighted what I have called the "internal" or upstream dimensions of biomedical boundary work by applying historical-professional and epistemological filters, respectively. Chapter 2 considered the *JAMA-Archives* theme issues as a network of profession-defining texts, in Bazerman and Paradis's terms, which I argued called forth a community of scholars wherein biomedical research on CAM was simply a routine matter. I showed that, although editors Fontanarosa and Lundberg claim CAM to be already well within biomedicine's purview, that claim was less descriptive than it was agenda-setting. CAM's legitimacy as an area of biomedical research was far from settled and remains to this day open to scrutiny. Drawing on Star and Bowker's research on classification, this chapter illustrated how biomedical studies of CAM in the 1990s set a course for future research by defining the practices that CAM comprises in essentially negative terms, as *not-biomedicine*. Emptied of their own internal significance, CAM practices are taken up in these medical journals within the framework of evidence-based medicine wherein, I argued, the randomized controlled trial functions, in part, as a technology of exclusion.

Chapter 3 applied an epistemological filter to biomedical boundary work by examining randomized controlled trials in CAM research. I argued that methodology operates in the *JAMA-Archives* theme issues as a rhetorical topos that can position research on CAM variously within and beyond biomedical boundaries, depending on a given commentator's orientation within the debate. I illustrated how the experimental article, as a genre, can persuade us to view biomedical research in terms that underemphasize the degree of variability involved in both the design of trials and the interpretation of their results. As a case in point, I isolated the concept of efficacy to show that, despite claims on all sides that the evidence on CAM will speak for itself, the notion of evidence itself can be marshaled persuasively in arguments about whether or not a given health intervention works. This is true, I illustrated, both in studies of CAM and in biomedical research more generally.

The fourth and fifth chapters moved from the medical profession to its points of contact with the public realm, applying clinical and public filters respectively. As Gieryn argues, while upstream science goes a long way to determine how science gets mapped as a bounded cultural space, the map itself depends crucially on reciprocal boundary work further downstream. Chapter 4 examined boundary work in the context of clinical practice. I argued that, because many commentators both within medicine and beyond cite CAM practices as attractive to patients because of their greater emphasis on practitioner-patient interaction, interaction itself can be a useful place to investigate how boundaries are configured by biomedical research on CAM. What I found was that practitioner-patient interaction is framed in trials of acupuncture and chiropractic primarily as a contaminant, as something to be controlled for through innovative design. I placed Burke's concept of terministic screens in relation to Arthur Kleinman's notion of explanatory models, which are defined as mental schemes for organizing and understanding illness and for making decisions based on those schemes. Putting Burke's and Kleinman's theories in relation to one another helped me to articulate a framework that could account for how interaction, and ideas about interaction, can persuade us toward different perspectives on how research on CAM ought to be conducted. I used the idea of placebo controls as a heuristic to show how the clinical trial model accounts for and contains the nonspecific and interaction effects of clinical encounters, which are often discounted as imaginary in research on CAM.

Popular media also play an important role in the downstream production and maintenance of medical boundaries; this was the "public filter" of chapter 5. I took as my example the 2002 *Newsweek* special report on biomedical CAM research, which announces, much like the *JAMA-Archives* theme issues, the arrival of a new, integrative model of medical research and practice. I examined the magazine as a cultural artifact and probed, first, the contours of the "new science" about which it reports, and then the conventional model of science that underlies it. I illustrated how the magazine, in parallel with the *JAMA-Archives* theme issues themselves, configures CAM research as both revolutionary and yet conventional and accepted by biomedical researchers and physicians.

I suggested in that chapter that one of the important features of popular reporting on CAM research is that the outcomes of CAM research are returned to the public that initially motivated the research. However, the sort of CAM that is returned to the public in *Newsweek* is both biomedicalized and implicitly hierarchical: while patients are drawn to CAM by its promise of greater patient agency and autonomy, the model of CAM that appears in *Newsweek*'s pages is thoroughly in the hands of the biomedicine. I argued, following Segal ("Breast Cancer"), that by reconfiguring CAM so fully within a biomedical framework, the story told in the *Newsweek* special report about the "new science" of CAM makes other stories about CAM harder to tell, such as stories about political, professional, and epistemic barriers to research on CAM and about how CAM practices are transformed as they are brought into the realm of biomedicine. Perhaps the most important story not told in *Newsweek*, I suggested finally, is a story about why so many patients are seeking so much health care to begin with, regardless of whether that care is mainstream, alternative, or "integrative."

In her review of scholarship in rhetoric of health and medicine, Segal argued that the "usefulness [of rhetorical projects on health] often lies in their ability simply to pose questions that are prior to the questions typically posed by other health researchers" ("Rhetoric of Health and Medicine" 228). The example she gives is of plastic surgery: while health research inquires about, for instance, how to make plastic surgery safer or about whether or not it should be reimbursable by insurance, a conceptually prior question would be about how "people [are] persuaded to see themselves as improvable by cosmetic surgery in the first place" (228). The question I raised at the end of chapter 5, about how so much medicine came to be necessary at all, was a similar sort of "prior" question. It is a question that underlies this book as a whole but one that I took up only indirectly. I return to it below, as I conclude, because it frames potential areas for future inquiry. First, however, I will expand on one of the prior questions that I did explicitly ask over the foregoing pages because this question can illustrate how, as I argued in my introduction, "the study of rhetoric at the fringes of medicine is illuminating for both medicine and rhetoric."

Throughout this book, especially in chapters 3 and 4, I examined how CAM interventions such as acupuncture and chiropractic fit (and do not fit) within contexts of biomedical research. As those chapters indicated, much health-related scholarship has focused on questions of how best to translate medical research into practice. (This, for instance, is one of the primary concerns of commentators within evidence-based medicine.) My own focus—my prior question—was instead on the models of practice presupposed in research contexts themselves. What can these models tell us about how we *conceptualize* medical practice—how we *think* medicine happens, as compared to how it actually does happen in clinics and hospitals? As chapter 4 explains, a rhetorical approach can articulate how different approaches to practitioner-patient interaction in research contexts can persuade: they can persuade us to view patients as particular kinds of decision makers, or to view medicine as unproblematically scientific, or to value some interventions over others. Biomedical boundaries can be negotiated in part through the ways that research accounts for practice.

A rhetorical approach illuminates what happens when patient-centered interventions are integrated into a system of medical practice that seeks to be essentially patient-free. Although research on doctor-patient interaction has consistently demonstrated the vital importance of the clinical exchange in patient care, this knowledge has not translated well into research contexts, where effects related to practitioner-patient interaction are often dismissed as statistical noise. The effort to purify health interventions of their contingency, their "noise," is in part rhetorical and boundary-focused: it constitutes an argument that draws lines of allegiance and of epistemic authority. For example, underneath the impulse to isolate spinal adjustment as chiropractic's "active ingredient" lie questions about allegiance to professional values, such as "What counts as an appropriate methodology?" and the corollary question, one of epistemic authority, "Who decides?" The challenges of placebo controls further open up to scrutiny the criteria for what qualifies as a contribution to knowledge.

The picture that emerged in my investigation of the models of practice effected in research contexts was one in which patients, in all their particularities, seem rather like statistical noise themselves. This observation is not new—it is a key idea behind many critiques of evidence-based medicine—but rhetoric adds texture to other critiques by offering a framework for tracing the slippage between conceptual models of medicine and the enactment of those models in research and practice.

This book contributes to health research by drawing attention to the persuasive element of biomedical research. While research produces invaluable knowledge about health and medicine, it simultaneously produces the professions that engage in it: biomedicine is ultimately recognizable *as* biomedicine because of its association with scientific methods and procedures. Boundary work is a constituent element of medical research because the ways that researchers line up their work with those methods and procedures will either assert the researchers' membership within the professional community or declare them outsiders. Consider, for instance, Fontanarosa and Lundberg's claim, as editors of the *JAMA-Archives* theme issues, that the articles on CAM published in the journals are unproblematically scientific because they were judged under the journals' "usual rigorous editorial evaluation and peer review" as conforming to the methods and procedures set by the biomedical community ("Call for Papers" 2112). Research on CAM, I have argued, is particularly well suited to the investigation of the rhetorical dimensions of biomedical research because the practices that CAM comprises do not fit easily with accepted scientific methods. Examining how such studies are designed and evaluated illuminates the persuasive aspects of biomedical research, generally, because the studies magnify the various contingencies that operate within it.

This book contributes to rhetoric by opening up a view on the means through which members of a culturally dominant profession respond to challenges to their jurisdiction while the profession appears, in effect, not to have been challenged at all. As the foregoing chapters have argued, the boundary work performed in the CAM-themed issues of *JAMA* and the *Archives* is virtually invisible, even as their authors air publicly their concerns about the potential impact of CAM research on their profession. Boundary conflict is part of the normal life of the professions as they compete for space within the professional ecosystem. But even if such conflict is normalized as routine in that ecosystem, that normalization does not account for the ability of the medical profession to engage in boundary work without appearing to have done so. Something about the rhetoric of boundary work covers its own tracks.

Examining this self-concealing aspect of the rhetoric of boundary work can return to rhetorical theory insight into processes that appear, on the surface, not to be rhetorical at all. While commentators on all sides of the biomedicine-CAM debate point to evidence produced by clinical trials as the key to settling where the boundaries of legitimate medicine ought to be, their own arguments about that evidence set boundaries, too. The study of these arguments can contribute to rhetoric a better understanding of, for instance, how boundary objects, such as the notion of efficacy, can both enable research across disciplinary borders and strategically draw lines of distinction among disciplines. Some boundary objects contain within them a degree of latitude that can be manipulated by dominant actors. They are, in other words, "rhetorically mobile."

The rhetorical study of biomedical boundary work can also enrich our understanding of how categories persuade by showing how residual categories can be invoked to lay claim over professional territory: by emptying the individual practices included in the category of CAM of their own particularities, the medical profession positions itself to overwrite them in biomedical terms. That is, as a "garbage" category, CAM is more easily reclaimed within a biomedical framework, or dismissed.

By way of conclusion, I would like to turn to a story that illustrates, in miniature, one of the larger claims I have made over the course of this book—a claim I framed in chapter 1 in Roy Porter's words, which bear repeating here: "quackery never prospers, for if and when it does, it becomes termed medicine instead" (207). Some years ago, I came across an article about the use of melatonin in child insomniacs on Babble.com, a website for trend-conscious urban parents. Author Cole Gamble reports that when his three-year-old daughter would not, or could not, sleep, an acupuncturist friend of his suggested trying melatonin, a hormone available in the United States as a dietary supplement. Gamble responded dismissively: "'Oh. Witchcraft.' This girl is nice, but she plans her week by astrological charts, so I tend to take her advice with a grain of not-crazy. I am not one for holistic medicine. I trust hard, pharmaceutical drugs with extensive clinical trials. If it hasn't been injected into a rat's eyeball or been ingested by thousands of monkeys, I can't take it seriously." Only when his friend explained that it was her pediatrician that led her to suggest melatonin did Gamble take her seriously and follow up with his own child's doctor, who agreed that melatonin might be worth a try. Gratified that the supplement came with the approval of the medical establishment, Gamble decided to give melatonin to his daughter and that night, she slept.

In the story of Gamble's daughter, we see first-hand how the clinical trial, as a research method, has accrued such rhetorical force that it is taken even in popular contexts to be "medicine's most reliable method for 'representing things as they really are'" (Kaptchuk, "Double-Blind" 541). The priority that Gamble accords to randomized controlled trials seems at first to contradict empirical findings that individuals seek CAM interventions without much regard to whether or not they have been successfully tested in clinical trials. Generally, this is true. However, what this example shows is how successfully CAM has been reframed, over the past two decades, within a biomedical framework.

Gamble's article was published in 2007, nearly a decade after the founding of the National Center for Complementary and Alternative Medicine (NCCAM) and the publication of the *JAMA-Archives* theme issues on CAM, and half a decade after *Newsweek* heralded the arrival of the "new science" of CAM. The efforts of these earlier discursive activities to expand biomedicine's boundaries to CAM seem to have been brought to fruition in Gamble's article. This is how he concludes: "All of my parenting efforts were nothing compared to that simple little pill. I can't help but feel a little powerless. But now that I sleep soundly and wake to a smiling, rested child, I think I can learn to live with this witchcraft in the pill bottle." In these lines, as in Gamble's article as a whole, the discourses of biomedicine and CAM are fused—or rather, CAM is described *in terms of* biomedicine. Gamble's disposition toward CAM and biomedical research illustrates the shift I have outlined over this book as the domain of biomedicine has increasingly expanded to other health care practices. As the various practices that constitute CAM are reframed in biomedical terms, they themselves become, in an important sense, biomedical.

The redescription of once-alternative health practices within biomedical terms was signaled, on a larger scale, by the renaming of NCCAM in December 2014 as the National Center for Complementary and Integrative Health (NCCIH). The center's director, Josephine Briggs, explained the change of name earlier that year in her call for public comment, in which she noted that "large population-based surveys have reinforced the fact that the use of true alternative medicine—that is, the use of unproven practices in place of treatments we know to be safe and effective—[is] rare." In this statement, Briggs takes the phrase "alternative medicine" to refer specifically to health interventions without any scientific evidence to support their use. Under this reasoning, practices such as acupuncture, which have produced mixed results in clinical trials, would count as alternative in some contexts and not in others. Briggs's primary concern was that inclusion of "alternative medicine" in the title of a National Institutes of Health-funded research center "may be misconstrued as advocacy or promotion of unproven practices." "Integrative medicine," by contrast, situates practices such as acupuncture, chiropractic, and herbal therapies squarely within biomedicine's boundaries.

NCCAM's transformation into NCCIH nearly twenty years after it was itself transformed from the Office of Alternative Medicine suggests that, although biomedical boundary work is ongoing, the specific rhetorical moment precipitated in the early 1990s by the push for scientific research on alternative medicine may be drawing to a close. For Briggs—as for the editors of *JAMA*, the *Archives* journals, and the *New England Journal of Medicine* before her—unorthodox health interventions that have not been demonstrated in clinical trials to be safe and effective should not be considered medicine at all, whereas interventions that originate "outside mainstream medicine" but are proven both safe and effective can and should be absorbed ("integrated") into biomedicine. Here, we see confirmation of Porter's observation that any unconventional health practice that prospers "becomes termed medicine instead." However, what I want to argue in closing is that the story of Cole Gamble's decision to try melatonin to help his daughter sleep illustrates not only that the domain of biomedicine has expanded to absorb nonbiomedical health practices. It also, more importantly, illustrates that biomedicine has expanded to absorb diverse other, nonmedical areas of human life.

To return to the implicit prior question that underlies this book, about why so many individuals are seeking so much health care (alternative and mainstream), I want, finally, to suggest that the story of Gamble's daughter is also a story of how a difficult and unsettling problem, such as a toddler's struggle to sleep, is redefined as a medical problem solvable with a pill. In this case, that pill is a dietary supplement, a CAM intervention that I argued in chapter 4 is rooted not in the idea of illness but of wellness. Whereas biomedical discourse often sets the terms of debate in an increasingly medicalized society, dietary supplements, as readily available commercial products, seem beyond medicine's reach. And yet, the idea of wellness itself—conceived broadly as *health maintenance*; contrasted with *illness treatment*—seems, paradoxically, to have the capacity to expand the domain of illness, bringing those who choose wellness-oriented products and services such as dietary supplements and other CAM practices into a realm defined instead by *dys*function. While these products appeal to individualist models of resistance against the so-called medical-industrial complex, the idea of wellness itself has been transformed into a new kind of dependence (this time, on supplements, handbooks, websites, consultants, and practitioners) that leaves its users resembling the disempowered, medicalized patients they seek not to become. "Wellness" has become, in effect, an illness-in-waiting, a transformation rooted in discourse that can be mined by rhetorical research.

Rhetorical analysis of biomedical boundary work can open up space for such study by isolating and describing the specific mechanics of the negotiation of borders between, for example, mainstream and alternative medicine, accepted and unaccepted methods and evidence, real and illusory treatment effects, and even between illness and health. Rhetoric at the fringes of medicine importantly determines what medicine is—and what it will be. The study of that rhetoric can consequently help us better understand how the notion of evidence can be mobilized to persuasive ends and how some health practices and practitioners come to and maintain ascendancy over others. By examining the means through which biomedical boundaries are effected through persuasion and are themselves persuasive, we also gain crucial insight into the means through which we come to know about our bodies and our health, and about our own place, as rhetorical subjects, in the realm of health and medicine.

Notes

Introduction

1. Lundberg was ostensibly fired for an unrelated but no less political matter—for publishing a report on Americans' definitions of sex that, according to the person responsible for firing Lundberg, American Medical Association executive vice president E. Ratcliffe Anderson, Jr., was keyed to the Bill Clinton-Monica Lewinsky scandal (Goldsmith; Horton). In an editorial condemning Anderson's decision, the *Lancet*'s editor-in-chief Richard Horton confirmed that Lundberg's "downfall" was widely believed to have been initiated by Lundberg's publication of the *JAMA-Archives* theme issues on CAM, which Horton says "caused the teeth of AMA officials to be ground heavily" (253).

2. In the chapters that follow, I examine definitions of mainstream and alternative medicine in detail but will note here that the category of CAM unites under a single rubric a disparate group of practices (e.g., chiropractic, energy healing, herbal medicine, homeopathy, meditation, naturopathy, traditional Chinese medicine)—a rubric that depends essentially on a negative relationship to conventional medicine. While the category of CAM is itself is problematic, its negative definition reveals how such practices are conceived, generally, in biomedicine: as not-biomedicine.

"Complementary" was added to "alternative medicine" during the mid-1990s. Complementary health practices are interventions used in conjunction with biomedical treatments, while alternative practices are interventions used in place of biomedical treatments (National Center). I discuss the more recent move toward the phrase "integrative medicine" in later chapters.

3. I use "deliberative" here in reference to the Aristotelian rhetorical occasion of deliberative rhetoric, a mode of discourse aimed at determining future policy or action.

4. While we cannot draw lines of causality between the *JAMA-Archives* theme issues and the later fortunes of complementary and alternative medicine vis-à-vis mainstream biomedicine, those fortunes indeed appear to have fallen since 1998. A recent survey from the US National Center for Health Statistics, for example, found a 50 percent drop in visits to CAM practitioners between 1997 and 2007, from 3,176 visits per 1,000 adults to 1,592 visits per 1,000 (Nahin et al.). Out-of-pocket expenditure for practitioner-based therapies also fell dramatically during that period, from an estimated $15.8–25.3 billion in 1997 (expressed in 2007 dollars) down to $11.9 billion in 2007 (Nahin et al.). Funding for the NIH's National Center for Complementary

and Alternative Medicine (NCCAM) also dropped off considerably several years after it was founded (National Center). Although NCCAM's annual budget doubled over its first three years (from $50 million in 1999 to $104.6 million in 2002), its budget increased only 4 percent annually between 2003 and 2005 ($114.1 million to $123.1 million) and has essentially flatlined ever since ($128.0 million in 2012, a gross increase of only 4 percent over 7 years).

5. Charles Bazerman, for example, shows how the experimental article stands as a "vicarious surrogate for the actual experiment" that persuades readers of the occurrence of events from which they are removed by both time and space (*Shaping Written Knowledge* 72). Similarly, Greg Myers argues that the processes through which scientific "texts produce scientific knowledge and reproduce the cultural authority of that knowledge" are deeply social and can be traced by studying documents such as draft and published versions of biology articles, grant proposals, and popularizations (*Writing Biology* ix).

6. Schuster, who formerly published under the name Mary Lay, illustrates how, in Minnesota in the mid-1990s, direct-entry midwives (lay-educated; contrasted with nurse-midwives) used licensing genres to assert jurisdictional claims over their area of practice—pregnancy and childbirth—and how those efforts nevertheless failed in the face of the greater institutional and professional resources of the biomedical community. Spoel has examined the rhetorical construction of midwifery as a profession ("Communicating Values," "Midwifery"; Spoel and James), focusing for example on the websites of two midwifery organizations in Ontario, Canada. Spoel argues that, despite the websites' description of midwifery as a communally oriented, woman-centered approach to pregnancy and childbirth, the professional ethos that those websites ultimately adopt "replicates more than it resists mainstream assumptions about the (non-communal) identities and relationships of health-care professionals and health-care publics" ("Communicating Values" 285).

7. Articles on rhetoric of health and medicine can be found in rhetoric and communication journals, such as *Rhetoric Society Quarterly*, *Quarterly Journal of Speech*, and *Technical Communication Quarterly*, as well as interdisciplinary journals such as *Journal of Medical Humanities* and *Social Science and Medicine*, and beyond. The Conference on College Composition and Communication (CCCC) has a newly established (2015) "Medical Rhetoric" Standing Group, after numerous years as a designated Special Interest Group, and the Association for Rhetoric of Science and Technology (ARST), which meets both at National Communication Association and Rhetoric Society of America, is likewise receptive to health and medical topics. Conferences further afield, such as the American Society for Bioethics and Humanities and the Society for Social Studies of Science, have also recently seen a strong showing in research in the area. See Segal for further reflection on these disciplinary groupings ("Interdisciplinarity" 312–15; "Rhetoric of Health and Medicine" 237–39).

8. "Conditions of possibility" in this quotation is drawn from Scott (*Risky Rhetoric* 21).

9. This study received institutional ethics approval and all names have been changed. Potential participants were identified by referral and through staff listings on clinic websites and were recruited via letter. Response rates varied: of the prospective participants initially contacted, both researchers, two of six TCM practitioners, and one of fifteen physician-clinicians offered to participate. A second, wider round of physician-clinician letters produced no further participants.

10. Other sample prompts: "Does the [study design/result] meet your expectations for a clinical trial?" (medical researcher); "Is this how most of your colleagues would treat this condition?" (TCM practitioner); "Do the results seem relevant to your own treatment of this condition?" (physician-clinician).

Chapter One

1. On audience design, see Clark and Carlson, who theorize the ways in which speakers "design their utterances" to situate their listeners as, variously, the persons directly addressed, members of the addressees' community, and overhearers (217). This "we" construction produces a defined community of addressees and simultaneously creates a category of not-addressed readers invited to "overhear" the conversations taking place in the journals. On identification and division, see Burke, *A Rhetoric of Motives*, 20–21.

2. See, respectively, "How to Brush Your Teeth," "The Science of Cooking," and "Evidence-Based Sports: Can a Team Have Too Many Star Players?"

3. An excellent primer on these questions is Wahlberg and McGoey's 2007 special issue of *BioSocieties* on EBM.

4. In the settlement of jurisdictional disputes, Abbott notes six possibilities: 1. *Full Jurisdiction*, where the profession claiming territory obtains it; 2. *Subordination*, where one profession occupies a position under the umbrella of another (e.g., nursing under medicine); 3. *Division of Labor*, with "functionally interdependent but structurally equal parts" (e.g., marriage counseling falling under the jurisdiction of psychiatrists, social workers, or clergy, among others; 73); 4. *Intellectual Jurisdiction*, where one profession's theory dominates but practice is assimilated among several (e.g., psychiatry's theoretical presence in other kinds of counseling); 5. *Advisory*, where one profession has some kind of influence over another, although that influence is not binding (e.g., the role of clergy in medicine); 6. *Workplace-Client Differentiation*, with less prestigious professions providing service to underserviced clientele (e.g., psychiatry treating wealthier patients; psychology, less wealthy ones; and social work, the poorest ones).

5. Physician Ronald Glasser critiques such an individualist-interventionist model of health care, arguing that "policymakers have consistently preferred the most expensive and least efficient models of health care, proving once again that the apostles of privatization are motivated not by hard-nosed economics but by an incoherent ideology that is little more than a brittle mask concealing the most irrational species of self-interest" (39–40).

6. In describing the marginalization of CAM in the *JAMA-Archives* theme issues as a *strategy*, I do not mean to imply that any individual authors necessarily or consciously planned to achieve a marginalizing effect. Rather, as I noted in the introduction, "Just as an organism might adopt a successful evolutionary strategy without being consciously aware of it, so too might an author adopt a successful rhetorical strategy without being consciously aware of it" (Ceccarelli, *Shaping Science* 5).

7. By "affective talk," I am referring to in-clinic conversations that do not relate directly to the patient's symptoms or treatment but relate, instead, to the patient's emotional well-being and his or her personal and work life. I discuss the affective dimensions of chiropractic care at length in chapter 4 but see also Oths, "Communication" and "Unintended."

8. The four trials on herbal supplements include Bensoussan et al.; Heymsfield et al.; Mc-Crindle, Helden, and Conner; and Melchart et al. The three acupuncture-related studies are by Cardini and Weixin; Shlay et al.; and White, Resch, and Ernst. The remaining studies are, respectively, Bove and Nilsson (chiropractic); Brent et al. (lanolin and breast shells); Garfinkel et al. (yoga); Hay, Jamieson, and Ormerod (aromatherapy); O'Connor et al. (relaxation); and Smolle, Prause, and Kerl (homeopathy).

9. Those two studies are Bove and Nilsson and Shlay et al. Bove and Nilsson are both doctors of chiropractic with biomedical PhDs and faculty appointments in medical schools (Harvard

and Odense Universities, respectively); Nilsson is also an MD. Shlay et al. coauthor Bob Flaws is a diplomate in acupuncture (DiplAc) and a well-known author and speaker on TCM.

10. This example is based on my own archival work on the Hughendon Collection, a Disraeli archive at Queen's University in Ontario. See also Kidd.

11. See Baer on bans against osteopaths and Villanueva-Russell on those against chiropractors.

12. Critics such as Kaptchuk and Kerr caution against uncritical acceptance of the "hagiographic history of the RCT," which canonizes the streptomycin trial as a revolutionary silver bullet in empirical research. Kaptchuk and Kerr argue that strategies against bias (blinding, randomization, etc.) were not "magically introduce[d]" to medicine by the new statistical sciences but have a long history stretching back centuries and, in some cases, even millennia (250). They rightly warn that celebratory, epideictic accounts of the streptomycin trial strip the randomized controlled trial of its complex social and political history.

13. I should clarify that my claim here is not that biomedical theory sponsors a one-size-fits-all approach to health care, or that CAM therapies are as individualized as their proponents suggest; these differences may be more apparent than real. See chapter 4 for discussion of the rhetoricity of models of practice in TCM and chiropractic.

14. The notion of evidence also performs gatekeeping functions in disciplines well beyond science and medicine, including in my own discipline of rhetoric and the related fields of writing/composition studies and technical communication (TC). In these fields, the methods through which knowledge is produced are tied directly to disciplinary status and identity, particularly as researchers have come under increasing pressure to grapple with "big data" in their studies (see Graham et al.). While the push toward generating ever-larger bodies of evidence in both medicine and rhetoric/writing studies/TC is driven by a will to expand and refine our store of knowledge in each field, the valorization of quantitative evidence in particular comes at the cost of other ways of knowing and restricts both the questions that researchers can ask and the methods available for answering them.

Commentaries on research methods in these fields generally turn on matters of disciplinary identity and prestige and intellectual autonomy. For surveys of these debates, which Berkenkotter has likened to "turf wars" (159), see Barton; Berkenkotter, "Paradigm Debates"; Charney, "Empiricism"; Goubil-Gambrell; Hansen; and McNely, Spinuzzi, and Teston. The combat-oriented, boundary-focused dynamics of such disputes are exemplified in Richard Haswell's searing critique of arguments against empirical research in writing studies, which were initially voiced in the late 1970s and early 1980s (Bizzell; Connors). Haswell and others such as Charney ("Empiricism"), Driscoll, and Driscoll and Perdue argue that resistance to empirical methods compromises the range and impact of research in the discipline because, in their view, only empirical methods meet the minimum standards of evidence in other academic disciplines.

The different positions exhibited in debates about methods in rhetoric, writing studies, and TC say as much about their proponents' intellectual and disciplinary commitments as about the actual quality of the scholarship, differences that run roughly along the lines of the humanities and the social sciences. However, these different allegiances are not incommensurable at all—indeed, they reflect the diversity of current scholarship on health and medicine within rhetoric, writing studies, and technical communication, which ranges from close textual criticism based on canonical rhetorical theory to analysis guided by genre theory, discourse analysis, and professional and technical communication, to observational and quantitative research. For an overview of the range of this research, see Segal's 2008 survey, "Rhetoric of Health and Medicine."

Critiques such as those cited here force scholars to consider carefully how research methods and the evidence they produce affect the delineation of boundaries even of their own disciplines. In rhetoric, as in biomedicine, the notion of evidence is loaded with rhetorical potential that can shift the boundaries between what counts as a valid contribution to knowledge and what does not.

15. I have cited the web version of the article. It was published in the hard copy magazine the following month under the name "When the Snake Oil Works" (*Atlantic* Oct. 2014: 26+).

Chapter Two

1. For upstream science, see, e.g., Latour; Myers, *Writing Biology*. For downstream science, see Charney, "Lone Geniuses"; Gieryn, *Cultural Boundaries*.

2. Epideictic rhetoric, one of Aristotle's three occasions or branches of rhetoric, is a ceremonial rhetoric of praise and blame, which aims to reinforce community values by celebrating those who exemplify those values, and making example of those who do not. Archetypal epideictic occasions include funeral orations and valedictory addresses.

3. Prominent journals that had published articles on complementary and alternative medicine prior to 1998 include the mainstream journals *JAMA*, the *Lancet*, and the *British Medical Journal* and CAM journals the *American Journal of Chinese Medicine* and *Complementary Therapies in Medicine*.

4. Charland's study of constitutive rhetoric examined the emergence in Québec in the early 1980s of the *peuple québécois*, a largely Francophone, sovereignty-seeking collective that, not existing previously, was brought into being through the publication of a 1979 policy document of the Province of Québec. The document advanced a case for Québec's independence from Canada, Charland argues, by framing this *peuple* as "oppressed" by the Canadian national government (216).

5. Here is Burke's quintessential definition of *identification*: "A is not identical with his colleague, B. But insofar as their interests are joined, A is *identified* with B. Or he may *identify himself* with B even when their interests are not joined, if he assumes that they are, or is persuaded to believe so. Here are ambiguities of substance. In being identified with B, A is 'substantially one' with a person other than himself. Yet at the same time he remains unique, an individual locus of motives. Thus he is both joined and separate, at once a distinct substance and consubstantial with another" (*A Rhetoric of Motives* 20–21).

Althusser explains that "*interpellation* or hailing . . . can be imagined along the lines of the most commonplace everyday police (or other) hailing: 'Hey, you there!'" Upon hearing this call, Althusser argues, "the hailed individual will turn round. By this mere one-hundred-and-eighty-degree physical conversion, he becomes a *subject*. Why? Because he has recognized that the hail was 'really' addressed to him, and that 'it was *really him* who was hailed' (and not someone else)" (174).

6. On rhetorics of "the people" in discourse surrounding the emergence of the *peuple québécois* in 1980s Québec, Charland argues that "not only is the character or identity of the 'peuple' open to rhetorical revision, but the very *boundary* of whom the term 'peuple' includes and excludes is rhetorically constructed: as the 'peuple' is variously characterized, the persons who make up the 'peuple' can change" (218).

7. I have excluded from this description of non-MD authors doctors of osteopathy (DO), whose training is akin to that of MDs but with an added focus on spinal manipulation that is similar to, but distinct from, chiropractic. Although DOs are often considered alternative

practitioners, they have had full practice rights on par with MDs since the 1960s. See Whorton, *Nature Cures*.

8. Edzard Ernst, MD, PhD, is another prominent CAM researcher that merits mention. Lead author of three articles in the theme issues and coauthor of two more, Ernst held the Chair in Complementary Medicine at the University of Exeter and is a prolific, outspoken critic of CAM. Now retired, he continues to publish widely in both scholarly and popular contexts on the need for more, higher-quality evidence of CAM's safety and efficacy, most publicly in his 2008 book *Trick or Treatment: The Undeniable Facts about Alternative Medicine* coauthored with Simon Singh (see Singh and Ernst).

9. All of the articles published in the theme issues underwent editorial review, although not all underwent external peer review. In *JAMA*, for instance, all articles published in the "Original Contributions," "Brief Report," "Health Law and Ethics," "On Call," and "Research Letter" sections are sent for external review, while articles in the "A Piece of My Mind," "Letters to the Editor," and "Commentary" sections are not. For my purposes here, I consider both sets of articles as peer-reviewed, insofar as they have all been evaluated in some form by colleagues within the same professional community.

10. In my early research for this book, I contacted *JAMA*'s editorial office to see if I could gain access, under conditions of confidentiality, to the peer review reports for the theme issues. My goal was to gain insight into the editors' and reviewers' criteria for including and excluding individual articles and for evaluating the studies' methods and results. The associate editor who responded to my query explained that my request was impossible to consider because confidentiality is foundational to peer review and medical publication. In a follow-up message, I clarified my proposed methods, including the study's provisions for confidentiality and their established precedence in writing studies research (in, e.g., Berkenkotter and Huckin), but no one at *JAMA* responded to my subsequent query.

11. Each of the *JAMA* theme issues on peer review were published in the year following their respective Congress on Peer Review, held in Chicago in 1989 and 1993, Prague in 1997, and 2001 in Barcelona. The subsequent theme issues were published on March 9, 1990 (*JAMA*, volume 263, issue 1), July 13, 1994 (272.2), July 15, 1998 (280.3), and June 5, 2002 (287.21). Regarding the outcome and impact of these congresses on peer review in biomedicine, *JAMA*'s deputy editor Drummond Rennie lamented in 2002 that, "Sixteen years after the [Congress on Peer Review] started, we find ourselves in the peculiar position of believing still more in the virtues of peer review, a system we know to be 'time-consuming, complex, expensive and . . . prone to abuse,' while we acknowledge that the scientific evidence for its value is meager" (2759–60; the quotation is from Drummond's own editorial in the 1998 peer review issue of *JAMA*).

12. For examples of how supporters of individual CAM practices adopt the CAM designation unproblematically, see, for instance, scholarly journals dedicated to CAM (e.g., *Evidence-Based Complementary and Alternative Medicine*, or *eCAM*), scholarly societies (e.g., Social Science Studies of CAM and Integrative Medicine), and patient handbooks (e.g., Mackenzie and Rakel, *Complementary and Alternative Medicine for Older Adults: A Guide to Holistic Approaches to Healthy Aging*), as well as professional organizations for CAM practitioners (e.g., European Federation for Complementary and Alternative Medicine, or EFCAM).

13. Off-label use is considered alternative in the Li study "because it does not conform to FDA regulations" (1449). The authors of the breast shell study, Brent et al., do not reflect on whether (and, if so, how) breast shells and lanolin constitute CAM but, in a sidebar, editor Catherine DeAngelis describes the intervention as a "self-administered, simple, natural" alternative to "more sophisticated and costly remedies" available to breastfeeding women (1077).

14. Happle advances twelve principles for the "epistemological demarcation" between "rational" (mainstream) and "irrational" (alternative) medicine that are worth listing in full: (1) alternative and regular medicine are speaking different languages; (2) alternative medicine is not unconventional medicine; (3) the paradigm of regular medicine is rational thinking; (4) the paradigm of alternative medicine is irrational thinking; (5) the present popularity of alternative medicine can be explained by romanticism; (6) some concepts of alternative medicine are falsifiable and others are not; (7) alternative medicine and evidence-based medicine are mutually exclusive; (8) the placebo effect is an important factor in regular medicine and the exclusive therapeutic principle of alternative medicine; (9) regular and alternative medicine have different aims: coming of age vs. faithfulness; (10) alternative medicine is not always safe; (11) alternative medicine is not economic; and (12) alternative medicine will always exist (1455).

15. The most accessed CAM practice in the 1998 Eisenberg study was relaxation, which I have excluded from my restricted definition of CAM because its popularity is not matched by correspondingly high levels of research. See Astin et al. on physicians' attitudes toward and patterns of referral to CAM.

Chapter Three

1. I thank one of my anonymous peer reviewers for the phrasing in the middle of this sentence.

2. In addition to the Cardini and Weixin and Shlay et al. trials, there is a third acupuncture trial published in the *JAMA-Archives* theme issues, White, Resch, and Ernst's trial of acupuncture for nicotine withdrawal in *Archives of Internal Medicine*. I focused on the first two trials only because I wanted to keep my discourse-based interviews under an hour and the first two trials feature the second and third largest participant populations of all RCTs in the *JAMA-Archives* theme issues (260 and 250, respectively, compared with White, Resch, and Ernst's at 76). Because larger trial populations generally allow for higher statistical power and greater sensitivity regarding treatment effects, the two larger studies seemed most likely to produce clinically significant results. In other ways, the Cardini and Weixin and Shlay et al. studies complement each other: Cardini and Weixin's trial was short, featured simple controls, was assessed by objective measures, and had a positive result, while Shlay et al.'s was longer, multi-armed, assessed subjectively, and negative.

3. Brecht's well-known "estrangement effect" is precipitated in dramatic performance by the collapse of the so-called fourth wall, the one separating performers from the audience. By collapsing this wall, Brecht contended, the theatrical illusion would be broken and viewers, unable to lose themselves within the fiction, would be forced to think critically about what they were seeing.

4. HRT had long been prescribed widely to menopausal women for prevention of heart disease and osteoporosis, based on data from several large, long-term observational studies, such as the Harvard Nurses' Health Study. Taubes estimates that, by 2001, some five million women took HRT preventatively. In 2002, however, the National Institutes of Health's Women's Health Initiative suspended its long-term RCT of estrogen and progestin, initiated in 1993, when participants in the intervention groups developed statistically significant higher rates of heart disease, breast and other cancers, stroke, and other negative outcomes (Writing Group). Millions of women stopped the therapy immediately. Since that time, the HRT tide has shifted several times and opinion is still divided as to its preventative effects and potential harms in different populations of women.

5. Systematic reviews are metastudies of RCTs. Typical evidence hierarchies can be found in Committee (97–98), Devereaux and Yusuf, and Grimes and Shulz.

6. It is worth noting that the systematic review is actually highest on the evidence hierarchy, as it produces metadata from multiple RCTs. However, in this chapter, I focus exclusively on the RCT because, as Feinstein and Horwitz point out, systematic reviews "can aggregate and evaluate but cannot change the basic information, [so] the RCTs themselves become the fundamental source to be considered both for quality and scope of data, and for the scope of topics contained in the EBM collection" (530).

7. The standardized acupuncture regimen, selected by a panel of eight acupuncturists, was based on the premise that the peripheral neuropathies caused by diabetes and HIV were similar; the points most commonly used for diabetes were then adopted. Patients experiencing other localized symptoms were additionally treated with supplemental points if they answered "yes" to the corresponding question. Both the depth and duration of needle insertion were standardized.

8. Pharmaceutical placebos are designed to look, smell, and taste like the investigational drugs so that the only real difference between them is the presence or absence of the drug under study. To Connolly, then, use of a control point that lacked the practitioner's *intention* would be the same as a using a placebo pill that was the wrong size or shape.

9. This initial presentation of the SAR as a new but uncontroversial textual entity fits with Segal's observation that, in medical journal articles, "Information is deemphasized in embedded structures; minor sentence elements reduce the effect of the information they contain—or imply the information is not new but given" ("Strategies" 527).

10. On genre appropriation, see, for instance, Bazerman ("Codifying") and Berkenkotter and Ravotas. Others, such as Schryer and Paré, have developed more stratified views of genre that explicitly address the movement of cultural capital through genre-use.

11. Published responses to the study's standardized acupuncture regimen (SAR) did not take issue with the authors' choice to standardize the procedure, although this may speak more to *JAMA*'s readership than to the idea of a SAR. Yet the fact that even the acupuncturists that responded in the journal to the study disputed only the particulars of the SAR, and not the concept of the SAR itself, suggests to me that even those familiar with acupuncture techniques realize the limits of what is permissible under the terministic screen of the RCT (see, e.g., Kaptchuk, Letter).

12. The view that writers working within the IMRaD structure simply provide "filler" for each "defined slot" was literalized by the 1996 publication of the first set of CONSORT (i.e., Consolidated Standards of Reporting Trials) guidelines, a twenty-two-item checklist for reporting trial results (Begg et al.). The most recent guidelines (2010) feature twenty-five items (plus subcategories), which require researchers to comment specifically on a study's blinding, randomization, outcomes measures, and other design features. See "CONSORT Statement."

13. For some of the earliest social-rhetorical critiques of replication, see Bazerman, *Shaping Written Knowledge*; Collins; Gilbert and Mulkay; Knorr Cetina; and Mulkay and Gilbert.

Replication serves similar argumentative functions in my own discipline of rhetoric and the related fields of writing/composition studies and technical communication. One might look, for instance, to debates about RAD research in composition, which Richard Haswell defines as "replicable, aggregable, and data supported." For Haswell, only RAD research on composition meets the minimum standards of evidence of other academic disciplines because, unlike "ephemeral" studies of writing that employ eclectic, individualized, and situation-specific methods, RAD studies are "enduring" because they allow other scholars to replicate their methods to test their conclusions, and to aggregate their results in future studies to extend them to new contexts (205). For Haswell, only RAD studies constitute "hard research" on writing (200, 214, 217), and are the only forms of research that can ensure the survival of rhetoric/composition as a discipline on the world stage.

Haswell's insistence on replicability as a means of bringing research on writing into alignment with (other) empirical disciplines is, of course, ironic: when Haswell advocated for RAD research in 2005, the notion of replication in the sciences had been known for two decades to function more rhetorically than epistemologically, serving as an assurance of careful research and affirmation of legitimacy rather than as a framework for the actual repetition and testing of earlier studies. The argument for replicable research in writing studies, then, seems to be at least partly a strategy of legitimation, to align research on writing with research in the sciences. For further discussion of replicability in writing studies research see Schryer; Swales.

14. This phrase is from Ian Hacking, whom Kaptchuk cites ("Intentional"), although Hacking is not himself writing on RCTs. On styles of reasoning, Hacking observes: "The truth is what we find out in such and such a way. We recognize it as truth because of how we find it out. And how do we know that the method is good? Because it gets at the truth" ("Statistical Language" 135). Kaptchuk argues that the same can be said for the RCT, which likewise authenticates itself through circular logic.

15. On cost-effectiveness, see Califf, who notes that "the idea that we pay more for a greater benefit is basic to most national economies. Yet in healthcare, there has been a tendency to expect that more effective therapies should save money. In fact, this is rarely the case" (429).

16. Jadad and Enkin, well-known authorities on RCT design, argue that "[b]oth efficacy and effectiveness approaches are reasonable and complementary" (15). See, also, Maguire, who examines the role of effectiveness studies in HIV research. He notes, for instance, that although efficacy is held up as the standard-bearer in FDA drug approval, effectiveness research was "legitimated" in 1989 as an acceptable means of data production, when aerosolized pentamidine became the first drug approved based only on community-based studies (80).

17. Of course, for some CAM skeptics, no level of scientific rigor will ever be enough. For example, Renckens insists that "The strongest attack [on biomedicine] arises when incomprehensible absurdities of alternative medicine are proven in impeccable trials" (531). See also Degele.

18. See, for instance, Abraham; Angell; Doucet and Sismondo; Dumit, *Drugs for Life*; Elliott; Healy; and Michaels.

19. Angell pinpoints the use of placebos to the 1962 Kefauver-Harris bill, which does not specify what drug manufacturers had to compare their products with to show efficacy. "It has since been taken literally to mean new drugs need not be compared with anything," she notes (286), since a placebo comparison would yield the strongest evidence of efficacy. Petryna points out that testing against placebo, while conventional in biomedical research, may actually violate the 2000 revision of the Helsinki Declaration of "Ethical Principles for Medical Research Involving Human Subjects," which asserts that new interventions ought to be tested against "the best current prophylactic, diagnostic, and therapeutic methods" (30).

Chapter Four

1. The Metaphor in End-of-Life Care (MELC) project, led by linguist Elena Semino at Lancaster University, is investigating how metaphors affect patients' experiences of death. Still in the preliminary stages, the research has found that although war metaphors invoking battles,

fighting, winning, and losing do work for some patients, those metaphors have negative effects on most patients. The researchers are preparing a "Metaphor Manual" for the UK National Health Service, to advise practitioners on how to select appropriate metaphors in caring for terminally ill patients ("Battle Metaphors"; Span). The previous examples of persuasion in clinical care in this paragraph are drawn from Derkatch and Segal.

2. The Canadian Institutes of Health Research (CIHR) comprises thirteen member institutes, including the Institutes of Aging, Cancer Research, Gender and Health, Musculoskeletal Health and Arthritis, and Population and Public Health. CIHR's research mandate aims to "strike a balance" among what it has identified as the "four pillars of health research": biomedical, clinical, health systems and services, and the social, cultural, and environmental factors that affect the health of populations (Canadian Institutes). Attention to the fourth pillar in particular, "social, cultural, and environmental factors," points to a shift to a more encompassing idea for health even in biomedical research contexts.

3. Incidentally, this definition is not far off from the ideal of evidence-based medicine. See, e.g., McCormack and Loewen.

4. The notion of the "lifeworld" comes from Mishler, who differentiated the "voice of medicine" from the "voice of the lifeworld," concepts that encompass, "respectively, the technical-scientific assumptions of medicine and the natural attitude of everyday life" (14).

5. Note that in both of these examples, which are Kleinman's own, the focus is doctor-centric: in the first case, the doctor must persuade the patient to view his or her condition within the limits of the biomedical explanatory model, while, in the second, the doctor must elicit the patient's own explanatory model as a means of securing his or her cooperation in medical treatment. Kleinman does not explore patients' persuasive potential as interlocutors, which may in part be a reflection of professional bias (he is himself a medical doctor, trained in psychiatry) but may also be the product of pragmatic assessment, on his part, of the weaker rhetorical position that patients occupy in medical contexts. The onus in his book, *The Illness Narratives*, is squarely on practitioners to effect changes within medical practice to the benefit of patients; patients themselves are afforded no such agency.

6. The quoted phrases in this sentence are from Oths, "Unintended" (107).

7. Perelman argues: "the aim of argumentation is not to deduce consequences from given premises; it is rather to elicit or increase the adherence of the members of an audience to theses that are presented for their consent. Such adherence never comes out of thin air; it presupposes a meeting of minds between speaker and audience" (9–10).

8. The Shlay et al. study described in the previous chapter combined sham controls and active controls in its three-armed study of acupuncture for HIV-related peripheral neuropathy.

9. See, respectively, Kaptchuk, "Placebo Effect"; Nahin and Straus; Brody and Miller; Finniss et al. and Kaptchuk, "Powerful Placebo"; and Hróbjartsson and Gøtzsche. ("Powerful").

10. Indeed, this is the goal of Harvard University's new Program in Placebo Studies and the Therapeutic Encounter (PiPS), founded in July 2011 under Ted Kaptchuk. Of its research program, the PiPS websites notes that

Just as evidence-based scientific research drives the progress of medical therapy, so too evidence-based research is needed to guide and enhance the art of medicine. Traditionally, the art of medicine has been understood as a humanistic orientation sequestered from medical science and technology. Research on the placebo response provides a fruitful opportunity for developing rigorous knowledge that can bridge this gap in the service of patient care. PiPS addresses this need by integrating concepts, research designs and analytic methods drawn from the clinical, basic and social sciences and the humanities. Our efforts are translational and cross-cultural. ("Research")

11. Ho and Bylund argue, for example, that although acupuncture operates on a holistic model of health (contra biomedical or biopsychosocial models), acupuncturists are split in adopting collaborative and paternalistic models of clinical interaction. This means that, although most traditional acupuncturists treat their patients as whole persons rather than treating them on the basis of individual symptoms, patients are often not accorded a significant role in making decisions about their own care.

12. It is worth noting that, by press time of the *JAMA* theme issue, the National Institutes of Health's Office of Alternative Medicine had been transformed into the National Center for Complementary and Alternative Medicine. The inclusion of the organization's former name and address appears to have been an oversight.

13. "Polyherbacy" derives from the term polypharmacy, which is defined as "excessive and inappropriate use of medications . . . resulting in an increased likelihood of adverse drug events, drug interactions, and . . . increased costs" (Nisly et al. 1).

Chapter Five

1. For critiques of the so-called dominant model of popular science in addition to Hilgartner, see Broks; Gross, "Roles of Rhetoric"; and Myers, "Scientific Popularization."

2. For recent surveys of rhetorical scholarship in public understanding of science, see Bell and Riesch, and Condit, Lynch, and Winderman.

3. The potential for individuals to be transformed through public discourse about health may be theorized, as Segal notes, as a function of what Ian Hacking calls the "looping effect," a process through which individuals become changed through their awareness of themselves as members of particular kinds or categories of people. "People of these kinds," argues Hacking, "become aware that they are classified as such. They can make tacit or even explicit choices, adapt or adopt ways of living so as to fit or get away from the very classification that may be applied to them" (*Social Construction* 34). This is the difference between *interactive* kinds, in Hacking's framework, and *indifferent* kinds, which are not so affected by their classification. To wit: "The classification 'quark' is indifferent in the sense that calling a quark a quark makes no difference to the quark" (105).

4. See, respectively, "Acupuncture Makes the Cover of Newsweek," "Newsweek Examines Back Pain," and "Newsweek Validates Complementary and Alternative Therapies for Back Pain."

5. I draw on articles published in other issues of *Newsweek* to illustrate how the report fits within the magazine's general coverage of CAM. I conducted an EBSCO search of *Newsweek* for the keyword "alternative medicine," which returned no hits before 1991 and 46 hits between 1991 and 2007. I read all of the articles returned in my search and included them as supplementary material in my analysis of the 2002 report. 30 percent of the hits in my search were from the special report, while the remaining articles align into two "peak" moments: the early 1990s (1991–1993), as CAM use began to rise and medical researchers first began to take notice, as evidenced by the 1992 formation of the Office of Alternative Medicine under the National Institutes of Health; and the late 1990s (1997–1999), when the *JAMA-Archives* theme issues were published and the Office of Alternative Medicine was transformed into the full-fledged National Center for Complementary and Alternative Medicine (NCCAM). These supplementary texts provide important context for the claims that the *Newsweek* report makes about the "new science" of CAM.

6. Presupposition, a concept from the linguistic subfield of pragmatics, refers to a proposition whose truth is taken for granted in a given statement. The magazine's opening question triggers a presupposition through the use of a wh- construction ("What is . . .") combined with a definite article (". . . the . . ."), which together presuppose or take for granted that there exists in the world a "real science of alternative medicine." Wh-questions include questions constructed using the "5 W's" (who, what, when, where, why) and other interrogatives such as "which" and "how." Levinson's well-known example of a wh-triggered presupposition is the question "Who is the professor of linguistics at MIT?" which presupposes that there is indeed a professor of linguistics at MIT (184).

7. I use the phrase "cover line" to align with magazine terminology, although Gudrun Held's phrase "text module" may be appropriate in terms of rhetorical theory, as it refers to groupings of text on magazine covers as persuasive units.

8. Political science, computer science, and Scientology are Randy Allen Harris's examples (Introduction, *Landmark Essays* xi); the others are my own.

9. On popular science as ready-made, see Calsamiglia and Ferrero; Fahnestock; Gross, "Roles of Rhetoric"; Michelle; and Schwartz, Woloshin, and Baczek.

10. The idea that successful rhetors must work within the value-systems of their audiences is as old as Aristotle, who contrasts the ease of praising "Athenians to an audience of them" with the daunting task of praising them instead to a crowd of Spartans or Scythians (51).

11. I am drawing here on Cassidy's discussion of Frank Turner's analysis of late nineteenth-century and early twentieth-century popular science texts, which Cassidy notes served to "argue the case for the legitimacy of science" in public culture (277).

12. For example, the standard "survivor narrative" tells us that we ought to be fearless and resilient as cancer patients, not to mention full of humor. To be otherwise, the narrative suggests, is a form of failure that can have not only social consequences but health consequences as well. Such narratives, Segal finds, imply that one's actual survival depends on one's performance of the role of "survivor."

13. For critiques of the so-called dominant view of popularization, see, for example, Bensaude-Vincent, Broks, Hilgartner, and Myers ("Scientific Popularization").

14. See, for example, Dumit (*Picturing Personhood*) on how brain imaging technologies shift how we think of our minds, as well as ourselves; Reiser on the influence of medical technologies on physician-patient relations; and Segal (*Health*) on how diagnostic technologies affect the rhetorical dynamics of medicine.

Notably, while we can clearly see in the artwork the individual cancer cells invading the body in Weiger and Eisenberg, and the exact vertebrae causing the problem in Cherkin, Sherman, and Eisenberg, the head depicted in Craig Miller's "Insight" on treatments for anxiety and depression is stubbornly opaque. The geometric x-ray reveals nothing but a lighter-colored portion of the same picture.

15. Note how often "doctor" is taken to denote authority of an unspecified sort. For example, Laura Schlessinger, who holds a PhD in physiology, uses the name "Dr. Laura" for her media work as a family and marriage counselor. Chiropractors and naturopaths also adopt the title in their professional designations, DC (doctor of chiropractic) and ND (naturopathic doctor).

16. Guiomar Ciapuscio's study of prepublication interviews between scientists and journalists provides a window into what is otherwise an invisible process. She notes that, when journalists gather information about the stories they write, "Scientists are always in charge of content presentation. . . . [with] the journalist merely ratifying, asking questions, demanding

explanations and nodding" (216). We could infer, from this process, the possibility that scientists' frameworks for thinking about the nature of their work might bleed into journalists' own frameworks for describing scientists' activities. Lewenstein suggests, also, that science writers have increasingly had formal scientific training, which may further contribute to shaping how journalists think about and describe science.

Conclusion

1. Here, again, is the key statement from the theme issues' editors, Fontanarosa and Lundberg: "There is no alternative medicine. There is only scientifically proven, evidence-based medicine supported by solid data or unproven medicine, for which scientific evidence is lacking" ("Alternative Medicine" 1618). For extended discussion of this passage, see the opening pages of chapter 1.

Works Cited

Abbott, Andrew Delano. *The System of Professions: An Essay on the Division of Expert Labor*. Chicago: U of Chicago P, 1988.

"About." *Evidence-Based Living*. Cornell University, n.d. Web. 5 July 2015.

Abraham, John. "Drug Trials and Evidence Bases in International Regulatory Context." *BioSocieties* 2.1 (2007): 41–56.

"Acupuncture Makes the Cover of Newsweek." *Acupuncture Today* 4.1 (2003): n.p.

Adler, Benard C. "Acupuncture." *Journal of the American Medical Association* 222.7 (1972): 833.

Agnew, Patricia A. *How to Talk to Your Doctor: Getting the Answers and Care You Need*. Sanger: Quill Driver, 2007.

Althusser, Louis. "Ideology and Ideological State Apparatuses." *Lenin and Philosophy, and Other Essays*. Trans. Ben Brewster. London: New Left Books, 1971. 127–88.

Anderson, Charles M. *Richard Selzer and the Rhetoric of Surgery*. Carbondale: Southern Illinois UP, 1989.

Angell, Marcia. *The Truth About the Drug Companies: How They Deceive Us and What to Do About It*. New York: Random House, 2005.

Angell, Marcia, and Jerome P. Kassirer. "Alternative Medicine: The Risks of Untested and Unregulated Remedies." *New England Journal of Medicine* 339.12 (1998): 839–41.

Aristotle. *The Rhetoric of Aristotle*. Trans. Lane Cooper. Englewood Cliffs: Prentice-Hall, 1932.

Ashcroft, Richard, Tony Hope, and Michael Parker. "Ethical Issues and Evidence-Based Patient Choice." *Evidence-Based Patient Choice: Inevitable or Impossible*. Eds. Adrian Edwards and Glyn Elwyn. New York: Oxford UP, 2001. 33–65.

Astin, John A. "Why Patients use Alternative Medicine: Results of a National Study." *Journal of the American Medical Association* 279.19 (1998): 1548–53.

Astin, John A., et al. "A Review of the Incorporation of Complementary and Alternative Medicine by Mainstream Physicians." *Archives of Internal Medicine* 158.21 (1998): 2303–10.

Baer, Hans A. *Biomedicine and Alternative Healing Systems in America: Issues of Class, Race, Ethnicity, and Gender*. Madison: U of Wisconsin P, 2001.

Barnes, Patricia M., et al. "Complementary and Alternative Medicine Use Among Adults: United States, 2002." *Advance Data* 343 (2004): 1–19.

Barry, Christine Ann. "The Role of Evidence in Alternative Medicine: Contrasting Biomedical and Anthropological Approaches." *Social Science & Medicine* 62.11 (2006): 2646–57.

Barry, Christine Ann, et al. "Giving Voice to the Lifeworld: More Humane, More Effective Medical Care? A Qualitative Study of Doctor-Patient Communication in General Practice." *Social Science & Medicine* 53.4 (2001): 487–505.

Barton, Ellen. "More Methodological Matters: Against Negative Argumentation." *College Composition and Communication* 51.3 (2000): 399–416.

"Battle Metaphors For Cancer Can Be Harmful." *Lancaster University*. 4 Nov. 2014. Web. 16 Nov. 2014.

Bazerman, Charles. "Codifying the Social Scientific Style: The APA Publication Manual as a Behaviorist Rhetoric." *The Rhetoric of the Human Sciences: Language and Argument in Scholarship and Public Affairs*. Eds. John S. Nelson, Allan Megill, and Donald McCloskey. Madison: U of Wisconsin P, 1987. 125–44.

———. *Shaping Written Knowledge: The Genre and Activity of the Experimental Article in Science*. Madison: U of Wisconsin P, 1988.

Bazerman, Charles, and René Augustín de los Santos. "Measuring Incommensurability: Are Toxicology and Ecotoxicology Blind to What the Other Sees?" *Rhetoric and Incommensurability*. Ed. Randy Allen Harris. West Lafayette: Parlor, 2005. 424–63.

Bazerman, Charles, and James Paradis. Introduction. *Textual Dynamics of the Professions: Historical and Contemporary Studies in Writing of Professional Communities*. Eds. Charles Bazerman and James Paradis. Madison: U of Wisconsin P, 1991. 3–10.

Beck, Rainer S., Rebecca Daughtridge, and Philip D. Sloane. "Physician-Patient Communication in the Primary Care Office: A Systematic Review." *Journal of the American Board of Family Practice* 15.1 (2002): 25–38.

Begg, C., et al. "Improving the Quality of Reporting of Randomized Controlled Trials: The CONSORT Statement." *Journal of the American Medical Association* 276.8 (1996): 637–39.

Begley, Sharon, and Debra Rosenberg. "Helping Docs Mind the Body." *Newsweek* 8 Mar. 1993: 61.

Bell, Alice R., and Hauke Riesch. "Researching Popular Science: More Diverse than the Limitations of Apparent Publishing 'Booms.'" *Public Understanding of Science* 22.5 (2013): 516–20.

Bensaude-Vincent, Bernadette. "A Genealogy of the Increasing Gap Between Science and the Public." *Public Understanding of Science* 10.1 (2001): 99–113.

Bensing, Jozien. "Bridging the Gap: The Separate Worlds of Evidence-Based Medicine and Patient-Centered Medicine." *Patient Education and Counseling* 39.1 (2000): 17–25.

Bensoussan, Alan, et al. "Treatment of Irritable Bowel Syndrome with Chinese Herbal Medicine: A Randomized Controlled Trial." *Journal of the American Medical Association* 280.18 (1998): 1585–89.

Berkenkotter, Carol. "Paradigm Debates, Turf Wars, and the Conduct of Sociocognitive Inquiry in Composition." *College Composition and Communication* 42.2 (1991): 151–69.

———. *Patient Tales: Case Histories and the Uses of Narrative in Psychiatry*. Columbia: South Carolina UP, 2008.

———. "The Power and the Perils of Peer Review." *Rhetoric Review* 13.2 (1995): 245–48.

Berkenkotter, Carol, and Thomas N. Huckin. *Genre Knowledge in Disciplinary Communication: Cognition/Culture/Power*. Northvale: Erlbaum, 1995.

Berkenkotter, Carol, and Doris Ravotas. "Genre as Tool in the Transmission of Practice over Time and Across Professional Boundaries." *Mind, Culture, and Activity* 4.4 (1997): 256–74.

Bishop, Felicity L., Eric E. Jacobson, Jessica R. Shaw, and Ted J. Kaptchuk. "Scientific Tools, Fake

Treatments, or Triggers for Psychological Healing: How Clinical Trial Participants Conceptualise Placebos." *Social Science and Medicine* 74.5 (2012): 767–74.

Bizzell, Patricia. "Thomas Kuhn, Scientism, and English Studies." *College English* 40.7 (1979): 764–71. Web. 2 Oct. 2014.

Blackwood, Bronagh. "Methodological Issues in Evaluating Complex Healthcare Interventions." *Journal of Advanced Nursing* 54.5 (2006): 612–22.

Blendon, Robert J., et al. "Americans' Views on the Use and Regulation of Dietary Supplements." *Archives of Internal Medicine* 161.6 (2001): 805–10.

Blumer, Ian. *What Your Doctor Really Thinks: Diagnosing the Doctor-Patient Relationship.* Toronto: Dundurn, 1999.

Booth, Wayne C. *The Rhetoric of Fiction.* Chicago: U of Chicago P, 1983.

Borgerson, Kirstin. "Evidence-based Alternative Medicine?" *Perspectives in Biology and Medicine* 48.4 (2005): 502–15.

Bourdieu, Pierre. "The Economics of Linguistic Exchanges." *Social Science Information* 16 (1977): 645–68.

Bove, Geoffrey, and Niels Nilsson. "Spinal Manipulation in the Treatment of Episodic Tension-type Headache: A Randomized Controlled Trial." *Journal of the American Medical Association* 280.18 (1998): 1576–79.

Bowker, Geoffrey C., and Susan Leigh Star. *Sorting Things Out: Classification and its Consequences.* Cambridge, MA: MIT P, 2000.

Bracken, Pat. "The Limits of Positivism." Letter in response to Kaptchuk et al. *British Medical Journal* 25.1 (2008): n.p. Web. 3 July 2009.

Brent, Nancy, et al. "Sore Nipples in Breast-feeding Women: A Clinical Trial of Wound Dressings vs. Conventional Care." *Archives of Pediatric Adolescent Medicine* 152.11 (1998): 1077–82.

Briggs, Josephine P. " Director's Page." www.nccam.nih.gov. 16 May 2014. Web. 25 Nov. 2014.

Britt, L. D., and Frederic J. Cole. "'Alternative' Surgery in Trauma Management." *Archives of Surgery* 133.11 (1998): 1177–81.

Brock, Bernard L., Robert L. Scott, and James W. Chesebro, eds. *Methods of Rhetorical Criticism: A Twentieth-Century Perspective.* Detroit: Wayne State UP, 1990.

Brody, Howard, and Franklin G. Miller. "Lessons from Recent Research About the Placebo Effect—From Art to Science." *Journal of the American Medical Association* 306.23 (2011): 2612–13.

Broks, Peter. *Understanding Popular Science.* New York: Open UP, 2006.

Bryant, Donald C. "Rhetoric: Its Functions and its Scope." *Quarterly Journal of Speech* 39.4 (1953): 401–24.

Burke, Kenneth. *A Grammar of Motives.* Berkeley: U of California P, 1969.

———. *Language as Symbolic Action.* Berkeley: U of California P, 1966.

———. *The Philosophy of Literary Form.* Berkeley: U of California P, 1973.

———. *A Rhetoric of Motives.* Berkeley: U of California P, 1969.

———. *The Rhetoric of Religion: Studies in Logology.* Berkeley: U of California P, 1970.

Burnham, John C. "The Evolution of Editorial Peer Review." *Journal of the American Medical Association* 263.10 (1990): 1323–29.

Bynum, W. F., and Roy Porter, eds. *Medical Fringe & Medical Orthodoxy, 1750–1850.* London: Croom Helm, 1987.

Califf, R. M. "Issues Facing Clinical Trials of the Future." *Journal of Internal Medicine* 254.5 (2003): 426–33.

Calsamiglia, Helena. "Popularization Discourse." *Discourse Studies* 5.2 (2003): 139–46.

Calsamiglia, Helen, and Carmen Lopez Ferrero. "Role and Position of Scientific Voices: Reported Speech in the Media." *Discourse Studies* 5.2 (2003): 147–73.

Canadian Institutes of Health Research. "Health Research Roadmap: Creating Innovative Research for Better Health and Health Care." *Canadian Institutes of Health Research*. Government of Canada, 22 Oct. 2009. Web. 29 June 2015.

Cardini, Francesco, and Huang Weixin. "Moxibustion for Correction of Breech Presentation: A Randomized Controlled Trial." *Journal of the American Medical Association* 280.18 (1998): 1580–84.

Carmichael, Mary. "Ginkgo on Your Mind?" *Newsweek* 2 Dec. 2002: 57.

Cassidy, Angela. "Evolutionary Psychology as Public Science and Boundary Work." *Public Understanding of Science* 15.2 (2006): 175–205.

Cartwright, Nancy. "Are RCTs the Gold Standard?" *BioSocieties* 2.1 (2007): 11–20.

Carver, Cynthia. *Patient Beware: Dealing with Doctors and Other Medical Dilemmas*. Scarborough: Prentice-Hall, 1984.

Ceccarelli, Leah. "A Hard Look at Ourselves: A Reception Study of Rhetoric of Science." *Technical Communication Quarterly* 14.3 (2005): 257–65.

———. "Manufactured Scientific Controversy: Science, Rhetoric, and Public Debate." *Rhetoric & Public Affairs* 14.2 (2011): 195–228.

———. "Neither Confusing Cacophony nor Culinary Complements: A Case Study of Mixed Metaphors for Genomic Science." *Written Communication* 21.1 (2004): 92–105.

———. *On the Frontier of Science: An American Rhetoric of Exploration and Exploitation*. East Lansing: Michigan State UP, 2013.

———. "Science and Civil Debate: The Case of E. O. Wilson's Sociobiology." *Rhetoric and Incommensurability*. Ed. Randy Allen Harris. West Lafayette: Parlor, 2005. 271–93.

———. *Shaping Science with Rhetoric: The Cases of Dobzhansky, Schrödinger, and Wilson*. Chicago: U of Chicago P, 2001.

Chalmers, Iain. "Unbiased, Relevant, and Reliable Assessments in Health Care: Important Progress During the Past Century, but Plenty of Scope for Doing Better." *British Medical Journal* 317.7167 (1998): 1167–68.

Charland, Maurice. "Constitutive Rhetoric: The Case of the *Peuple Québécois*." *Landmark Essays in Rhetorical Criticism*. Ed. Thomas W. Benson. Davis: Hermagoras, 1993. 213–34.

Charney, Davida. "Empiricism Is Not a Four-Letter Word." *College Composition and Communication* 47.4 (1996): 567–93. Web. 3 Oct. 2014.

———. "Introduction: The Rhetoric of Popular Science." *Written Communication* 21.1 (2004): 3–5.

———. "Lone Geniuses in Popular Science: The Devaluation of Scientific Consensus." *Written Communication* 20.3 (2003): 215–41.

Cherkin, Dan, Karen Sherman, and David Eisenberg. "Beyond the Backache." *Newsweek* 2 Dec. 2002: 56.

Ciapuscio, Guiomar E. "Formulation and Reformulation Procedures in Verbal Interactions between Experts and (Semi-)Laypersons." *Discourse Studies* 5.2 (2003): 207–33.

Cicourel, Aaron V. "The Reproduction of Objective Knowledge: Common Sense Reasoning in Medical Decision Making." *The Knowledge Society*. Eds. Gernot Böhme and Nico Stehr. Boston: D. Reidel, 1986. 87–122.

Cirigliano, Michael, and Anthony Sun. "Advising Patients About Herbal Therapies." *Journal of the American Medical Association* 280.18 (1998): 1565–66.

Clark, Herbert H., and Thomas B. Carlson. "Hearers and Speech Acts." *Arenas of Language Use.* Chicago: U of Chicago P, 1992. 205–47.

Collins, Harry. *Changing Order: Replication and Induction in Scientific Practice.* Chicago: University of Chicago P, 1985.

Committee on the Use of Complementary and Alternative Medicine by the American Public, Board on Health Promotion and Disease Prevention, Institute of Medicine of the National Academies. *Complementary and Alternative Medicine in the United States.* Washington, DC: The National Academies, 2005.

Condit, Celeste M., John Lynch, and Emily Winderman. "Recent Rhetorical Studies in Public Understanding of Science." *Public Understanding of Science* 21.4 (2013): 386–400.

Connors, Robert J. "Composition and Science." *College English* 45.1 (1983): 1–20. Web. 2 Oct. 2014.

Conrad, Peter. *The Medicalization of Society: On the Transformation of Human Conditions into Treatable Disorders.* Baltimore: Johns Hopkins UP, 2007.

"CONSORT Statement." *Consort: Transparent Reporting of Trials.* 20 Jan. 2012. Web. 25 Feb. 2014.

Cowley, Geoffrey. "Now 'Integrative' Care." *Newsweek* 2 Dec. 2002: 46.

Cowley, Geoffrey, and Anne Underwood. "What's 'Alternative'?" *Newsweek* 23 Nov. 1998: 68.

Daaleman, Timothy P., and Bruce Frey. "Prevalence and Patterns of Physician Referral to Clergy and Pastoral Care Providers." *Archives of Family Medicine* 7.6 (1998): 548–53.

Dalen, James E. " 'Conventional' and 'Unconventional' Medicine: Can They Be Integrated?" *Archives of Internal Medicine* 158.20 (1998): 2179–81.

Dascal, Marcelo, and Alan G. Gross. "The Marriage of Pragmatics and Rhetoric." *Philosophy and Rhetoric* 32.2 (1999): 107–30.

DeAngelis, Catherine D. Editor's response to Demetrios Theodoropoulos. *Archives of Pediatric Adolescent Medicine* 152.6 (1998): 606.

DeAngelis, Catherine D., and Phil B. Fontanarosa. "Drugs Alias Dietary Supplements." *Journal of the American Medical Association* 290.11 (2003): 1519–20.

Degele, Nina. "On the Margins of Everything: Doing, Performing, and Staging Science in Homeopathy." *Science, Technology, and Human Values* 30.1 (2005): 111–36.

deGrasse Tyson, Neil (neiltyson). "Q: What do you call Alternative Medicine that survives double-blind laboratory tests? A: Regular Medicine." 30 May 2012, 22:12. https://twitter.com /neiltyson/status/208063372200128512. Tweet.

Delbanco, Thomas L. "Leeches, Spiders, and Astrology: Predilections and Predictions." *Journal of the American Medical Association* 280.18 (1998): 1560–62.

Denis, Jean-Louis, et al. "Explaining Diffusion Patterns for Complex Health Care Innovations." *Health Care Management Review* 27.3 (2002): 60–73.

de Oliveira, Janaina Minelli, and Adriana Silvina Pagano. "The Research Article and the Science Popularization Article: A Probabilistic Functional Grammar Perspective on Direct Discourse Representation." *Discourse Studies* 8.5 (2006): 627–46.

Derkatch, Colleen. " 'Wellness' as Incipient Illness: Dietary Supplement Discourse in a Biomedical Culture." *Present Tense: A Journal of Rhetoric in Society* 2.2 (2012): n.p.

Derkatch, Colleen, and Judy Z. Segal. "Realms of Rhetoric in Health and Medicine." *University of Toronto Medical Journal* 82.2 (2005): 138–142.

Devereaux, P. J., and S. Yusuf. "The Evolution of the Randomized Controlled Trial and its Role in Evidence-Based Decision Making." *Journal of Internal Medicine* 254.2 (2003): 105–13.

Dieppe, Paul. "Trial Designs and Exploration of the Placebo Response." *Complementary Therapies in Medicine* 21 (2013): 105–108.

Dopson, Sue, et al. "No Magic Targets! Changing Clinical Practice To Become More Evidence Based." *Health Care Management Review* 27.3 (2002): 35–47.

Doucet, Mathieu, and Sergio Sismondo. "Evaluating Solutions to Sponsorship Bias." *Journal of Medical Ethics* 34 (2008): 627–30.

Dowdey, Diane. "Rhetorical Techniques of Audience Adaptation in Popular Science Writing." *Journal of Technical Writing and Communication* 17.3 (1987): 275–85.

Driscoll, Dana Lynn. "Composition Studies, Professional Writing and Empirical Research: A Skeptical View." *Journal of Technical Writing and Communication* 39.2 (2009): 195–204. Web. 3 Oct. 2014.

Driscoll, Dana, and Sherry Wynn Perdue. "Theory, Lore, and More: Analysis of RAD Research in *The Writing Center Journal*, 1980–2009." *Writing Center Journal* 32.1 (2012): 11–39.

Dumit, Joseph. *Drugs for Life: How Pharmaceutical Companies Define Our Health.* Durham: Duke UP, 2012.

———. *Picturing Personhood: Brain Scans and Biomedical Identity.* Princeton: Princeton UP, 2004.

Edwards, Adrian, and Glyn Elwyn, eds. *Evidence-based Patient Choice: Inevitable or Impossible?* New York: Oxford UP, 2001.

Eisenberg, David M., et al. "Trends in Alternative Medicine Use in the United States, 1990–1997: Results of a Follow-Up National Survey." *Journal of the American Medical Association* 280.18 (1998): 1569–75.

Eisenberg, David M., et al. "Unconventional Medicine in the United States: Prevalence, Costs, and Patterns of Use." *New England Journal of Medicine* 328.4 (1993): 246–52.

Elliott, Carl. *White Coat, Black Hat: Adventures on the Dark Side of Medicine.* Boston: Beacon, 2010.

Elpern, David J. "Beyond Complementary and Allopathic Medicine." *Archives of Dermatology* 134.11 (1998): 1473–76.

Elwyn, Glyn, and Adrian Edwards. "Evidence-Based Patient Choice?" *Evidence-Based Patient Choice: Inevitable or Impossible?* Eds. Adrian Edwards and Glyn Elwyn. New York: Oxford UP, 2001. 3–18.

Emmons, Kimberly K. *Black Dogs and Blue Words: Depression and Gender in the Age of Self-Care.* New Brunswick: Rutgers UP, 2010.

Enck, Paul, et al. "The Placebo Response in Medicine: Minimize, Maximize or Personalize?" *Nature Reviews Drug Discovery* 13.3 (2013): 191–204.

Ente, Gerald. Letter in response to Demetrios Theodoropoulos. *Archives of Pediatric Adolescent Medicine* 152.11 (1998): 1154.

Epstein, Ronald M., et al. "Measuring Patient-Centered Communication in Patient-Physician Consultations: Theoretical and Practical Issues." *Social Science & Medicine* 61.7 (2005): 1516–28.

Ernst, Edzard, and Max H. Pittler. "Efficacy of Homeopathic Arnica: A Systematic Review of Placebo-Controlled Clinical Trials." *Archives of Surgery* 133.11 (1998): 1187–90.

Ernst, Edzard, Julia I. Rand, and Clare Stevinson. "Complementary Therapies for Depression: An Overview." *Archives of General Psychiatry* 55.11 (1998): 1026–32.

Ernst, Edzard, and Adrian R. White. "Acupuncture for Back Pain: A Meta-Analysis of Randomized Controlled Trials." *Archives of Internal Medicine* 158.20 (1998): 2235–41.

Evans, Robert. "Introduction: Demarcation Socialized: Constructing Boundaries and Recognizing Difference." *Science, Technology, and Human Values* 30.1 (2005): 3–16.

Evidence-Based Living. Cornell University, n.d. Web. 5 July 2015.

Evidence-Based Medicine Working Group. "Evidence-Based Medicine: A New Approach to Teaching the Practice of Medicine." *Journal of the American Medical Association* 268.17 (1992): 2420–25.

"Evidence-Based Sports: Can a Team Have Too Many Star Players?" *Evidence-Based Living.* Cornell University, n.d. Web. 5 July 2015.

Ezzo, Jeanette, et al. "Complementary Medicine and the Cochrane Collaboration." *Journal of the American Medical Association* 280.18 (1998): 1628–30.

Fahnestock, Jeanne. "Accommodating Science: The Rhetorical Life of Scientific Facts." *Written Communication* 15.3 (1998): 330–50.

———. "Preserving the Figure: Consistency in the Presentation of Scientific Arguments." *Written Communication* 21.1 (2004): 6–31.

Feinstein, Alvan R., and Ralph I. Horwitz. "Problems in the 'Evidence' of 'Evidence-Based Medicine.'" *American Journal of Medicine* 103.6 (1997): 529–35.

Fergusson, Dean, et al. "Turning a Blind Eye: The Success of Blinding Reported in a Random Sample of Randomised, Placebo Controlled Trials." *British Medical Journal* 328.432 (2004): n.p. Web. 26 Aug. 2005.

Feyerabend, Paul K. *Against Method: Outline of an Anarchistic Theory of Knowledge.* London: Verso, 1993.

Finniss, Damien G., et al. "Biological, Clinical, and Ethical Advances of Placebo Effects." *Lancet* 375.9715 (2010): 686–95.

Firenzuoli, Fabio, and Luigi Gori. "Evidence Based Medicine as Frame of Phytotherapy." Letter in response to Sackett et al. *British Medical Journal* (15 Aug. 2000): n.p. Web. 26 June 2009.

Fontanarosa, Phil B., ed. *Alternative Medicine: An Objective Assessment.* Chicago: American Medical Association, 2000.

Fontanarosa, Phil B., and George D. Lundberg. "Alternative Medicine Meets Science." *Journal of the American Medical Association* 280.18 (1998): 1618–19.

———. "Complementary, Alternative, Unconventional, and Integrative Medicine: Call for Papers for the Annual Coordinated Theme Issues of the AMA Journals." *Journal of the American Medical Association* 278.23 (1997): 2111–12.

Fontenot, Sarah Freymann. "PCORI, Comparative Effectiveness and the ACA: Improving Patient Outcomes or Cookbook Medicine?" *Physician Executive* 39.4 (2013): 98–102.

Ford, Sarah, Theo Schofield, and Tony Hope. "What are the Ingredients for a Successful Evidence-Based Patient Choice Consultation? A Qualitative Study." *Social Science & Medicine* 56.3 (2003): 589–602.

Foss, Sonja K. *Rhetorical Criticism: Exploration and Practice.* Prospect Heights: Waveland, 1989.

Foucault, Michel. *The Birth of the Clinic: An Archaeology of Medical Perception.* Trans. Alan Sheridan. New York: Routledge, 2003.

Frankel, Richard, and Howard Beckman. "Evaluating the Patient's Primary Problem(s)." *Communicating with Medical Patients.* Eds. Moira Stewart and Debra Roter. London: Sage, 1989. 86–98.

Fujimura, Joan H. "Crafting Science: Standardized Packages, Boundary Objects, and 'Translation.'" *Science as Practice and Culture.* Ed. Andrew Pickering. Chicago: U of Chicago P, 1992. 168–214.

Galison, Peter Louis. *Image and Logic: A Material Culture of Microphysics.* Chicago: U of Chicago P, 1997.

Gamble, Cole. "Saved by the Pill." *Babble.* 4 Oct. 2007. Web. 20 Aug. 2009.

Garfinkel, Marian S., et al. "Yoga-Based Intervention for Carpal Tunnel Syndrome: A Randomized Trial." *Journal of the American Medical Association* 280.18 (1998): 1601–03.

Garges, Harmony P., Indu Varia, and P. Murali Doraiswamy. "Cardiac Complications and Delirium Associated with Valerian Root Withdrawal." *Journal of the American Medical Association* 280.18 (1998): 1566–67.

Gevitz, Norman. "'A Coarse Sieve': Basic Science Boards and Medical Licensure in the United States." *Journal of the History of Medicine and Allied Sciences* 43 (1988): 36–63.

Gieryn, Thomas F. "Boundary-Work and the Demarcation of Science from Non-Science: Strains and Interests in Professional Ideologies of Scientists." *American Sociological Review* 48.6 (1983): 781–95.

———. *Cultural Boundaries of Science: Credibility on the Line.* Chicago: U of Chicago P, 1999.

Gilbert, G. Nigel, and Michael Mulkay. *Opening Pandora's Box: A Sociological Analysis of Scientists' Discourse.* New York: Cambridge UP, 1984.

Giltrow, Janet. "Genre and the Pragmatic Concept of Background Knowledge." *Genre and the New Rhetoric.* Eds. Aviva Freedman and Peter Medway. London: Taylor and Francis, 1995. 155–78.

———. "Modern Conscience: Modalities of Obligation in Research Genres." *Text* 25.2 (2005): 171–99.

Glasser, Ronald J. "We Are Not Immune: Influenza, SARS, and the Collapse of Public Health." *Harper's.* July 2004: 35–42.

Glick, Daniel. "New Age Meets Hippocrates." *Newsweek* 13 July 1992: 58.

Goldacre, Ben, and Carl Heneghan. "How Medicine Is Broken, And How We Can Fix It." *British Medical Journal* 350 (2015): n.p.

Goldsmith, Marsha F. "George D. Lundberg Ousted as *JAMA* Editor." *Journal of the American Medical Association* 281.5 (1999): 403.

Goodwin, James S., and Michael R. Tangum. "Battling Quackery: Attitudes about Micronutrient Supplements in American Academic Medicine." *Archives of Internal Medicine* 158.20 (1998): 2187–91.

Gorman, Michael E. "Levels of Expertise and Trading Zones: A Framework for Multidisciplinary Collaboration." *Social Studies of Science* 32.5/6 (2002): 933–38.

Goubil-Gambrell, Patricia. "Guest Editor's Column." *Technical Communication Quarterly* 7.1 (1998): 5–7. Web. 5 Oct. 2014.

Graham, S. Scott. *The Politics of Pain Medicine: A Rhetorical-Ontological Inquiry.* Chicago: U Chicago P, 2015.

Graham, S. Scott, et al. "Statistical Genre Analysis: Toward Big Data Methodologies in Technical Communication." *Technical Communication Quarterly* 24.1 (2015): 70–104.

Grant, Kelly. "Pioneering Ontario Clinic Hopes to Make Naturopathy Mainstream." *Globe and Mail* 25 Feb. 2014. Web. 23 Mar. 2014.

Grimes, David A., and Kenneth F. Schulz. "An Overview of Clinical Research: The Lay of the Land." *Lancet* 359.9300 (2002): 57–61.

Gross, Alan G. "Persuasion and Peer Review in Science: Habermas's Ideal Speech Situation Applied." *History of the Human Sciences* 3.2 (1990): 195–209.

———. *The Rhetoric of Science.* Cambridge: Harvard UP, 1990.

———. "The Roles of Rhetoric in the Public Understanding of Science." *Public Understanding of Science* 3.1 (1994): 3–23.

Gülich, Elisabeth. "Conversational Techniques Used in Transferring Knowledge between Medical Experts and Non-experts." *Discourse Studies* 5.2 (2003): 235–63.

Hacking, Ian. *The Social Construction of What?* Cambridge: Harvard UP, 1999.

———. "Statistical Language, Statistical Truth and Statistical Reason: The Self-Authentification of a Style of Scientific Reasoning." *The Social Dimensions of Science*. Ed. Ernan McMullin. Notre Dame: U of Notre Dame P, 1992. 130–57.

Hamblin, James. "There Is No 'Alternative Medicine.'" *The Atlantic.com*. Atlantic Monthly Group, 17 Sept. 2014. Web. 3 July 2015.

Hamer, Pamela. "Animal Acupuncture." *Newsweek* 20 Dec. 2004: 10.

Hamilton, Kendall. "Reaching for the Rock." *Newsweek* 20 Jan. 1997: 48.

Hansen, Kristine. "Are We There Yet? The Making of a Discipline in Composition." *Changing of Knowledge in Composition: Contemporary Perspectives*. Eds. Lance Massey and Richard Gebhardt. Logan: Utah State UP, 2011. 236–63.

Happle, Rudolf. "The Essence of Alternative Medicine: A Dermatologist's View from Germany." *Archives of Dermatology* 134.11 (1998): 1455–60.

Harris, Randy Allen. Introduction. *Landmark Essays on Rhetoric of Science: Case Studies*. Ed. Randy Allen Harris. Mahwah: Hermagoras, 1997. xi–xlv.

———. Introduction. *Rhetoric and Incommensurability*. Ed. Randy Allen Harris. West Lafayette: Parlor, 2005. 3–149.

———. "Reception Studies in the Rhetoric of Science." *Technical Communication Quarterly* 14.3 (2005): 249–55.

Haskell, William, and David Eisenberg. "Ways to Heal Your Heart." *Newsweek* 2 Dec. 2002: 52.

Haswell, Richard. "NCTE/CCCC's Recent War on Scholarship." *Written Communication* 22.2 (2005): 198–223. Web. 2 Oct. 2014.

Hay, Isabelle C., Margaret Jamieson, and Anthony D. Ormerod. "Randomized Trial of Aroma-therapy: Successful Treatment For Alopecia Areata." *Archives of Dermatology* 134.11 (1998): 1349–52.

Healy, David. *Pharmageddon*. Berkeley: U of California P, 2012.

Heifferon, Barbara, and Stuart C. Brown, eds. *Rhetoric of Healthcare: Essays Toward A New Disciplinary Inquiry*. Cresskill: Hampton, 2008.

Held, Gudrun. "Magazine Covers: A Multimodal Pretext-Genre." *Folia Linguistica* 39.1/2 (2005): 173–96.

Held, P., H. Wedel, and L. Wilhelmsen. "Clinical Trials: Introduction." *Journal of Internal Medicine* 254.2 (2003): 103–04.

Henwood, Flis, Roma Harris, and Philippa Spoel. "Informing Health? Negotiating theLogics of Choice and Care in Everyday Practices of 'Healthy Living.'" *Social Science and Medicine* 12 (2011): 2026–32.

Heymsfield, Steven B., et al. "*Garcinia cambogia* (Hydroxycitric Acid) as a Potential Antiobesity Agent: A Randomized Controlled Trial." *Journal of the American Medical Association* 280.18 (1998): 1596–1600.

Hilgartner, Stephen. "The Dominant View of Popularization: Conceptual Problems, Political Uses." *Social Studies of Science* 20.3 (1990): 519–39.

Ho, Evelyn Y. "Behold the Power of Qi: The Importance of Qi in the Discourse of Acupuncture." *Research on Language & Social Interaction* 39.4 (2006): 411–40.

Ho, Evelyn Y., and Carma L. Bylund. "Models of Health and Models of Interaction in the Practitioner-Client Relationship in Acupuncture." *Health Communication* 23.6 (2008): 506–15.

Horrobin, David F. "Philosophical Basis of Peer Review and the Suppression of Innovation." *Journal of the American Medical Association* 263.10 (1990): 1438–41.

Horton, Richard. "The Sacking of JAMA." *Lancet* 353.9149 (1999): 252–53.

"How to Brush Your Teeth." *Evidence-Based Living*. Cornell University, n.d. Web. 5 July 2015.

Hróbjartsson, Asbjorn, and Peter C. Gøtzsche. "Is the Placebo Powerless? An Analysis of Clinical Trials Comparing Placebo with No Treatment." *New England Journal of Medicine* 344.21 (2001): 1594–1602.

Hsu, Dora T., and David L. Diehl. "Acupuncture: The West Gets the Point." *Lancet* 352 Suppl. 4 (1998): SIV1.

Hunter, Kathryn Montgomery. *Doctors' Stories: The Narrative Structure of Medical Knowledge*. Princeton: Princeton UP, 1991.

Hwang, Mi Young. "Alternative Choices: What it Means to Use Nonconventional Medical Therapy [*JAMA* Patient Page]." *Journal of the American Medical Association* 280.18 (1998): 1640.

International Committee of Medical Journal Editors. "Preparing for Submission." www.icmje .org. n.d. Web. 25 Feb. 2014.

Jacobs, Jennifer, Edward H. Chapman, and Dean Crothers. "Patient Characteristics and Practice Patterns of Physicians Using Homeopathy." *Archives of Family Medicine* 7.6 (1998): 537–40.

Jadad, Alejandro R., and Murray Enkin. *Randomized Controlled Trials: Questions, Answers, and Musings*. Malden: Blackwell, 2007.

Jensen, Uffe Juul. "The Struggle for Clinical Authority: Shifting Ontologies and the Politics of Evidence." *BioSocieties* 2.1 (2007): 101–14.

Jonas, Wayne B. "Alternative Medicine—Learning from the Past, Examining the Present, Advancing to the Future." *Journal of the American Medical Association* 280.18 (1998): 1616–18.

Journet, Debra. "Interdisciplinary Discourse and 'Boundary Rhetoric': The Case of S. E. Jelliffe." *Written Communication* 10.4 (1993): 510–41.

Jüni, Peter, et al. "The Hazards of Scoring the Quality of Clinical Trials for Meta-Analysis." *Journal of the American Medical Association* 282.11 (1999): 1054–60.

Jutel, Annemarie Goldstein. *Putting a Name to It: Diagnosis in Contemporary Society*. Baltimore: Johns Hopkins UP, 2011.

Kalb, Claudia. "How to Lift The Mind." *Newsweek* 2 Dec. 2002: 67.

———. "A Natural Way to Age." *Newsweek* 2 Dec. 2002: 64.

Kaptchuk, Ted. Authors' response to Kaptchuk et al. *British Medical Journal* 25.1 (2008): n.p. Web. 1 Aug. 2009.

———. "The Double-Blind, Randomized, Placebo-Controlled Trial: Gold Standard or Golden Calf?" *Journal of Clinical Epidemiology* 54.6 (2001): 541–49.

———. "Intentional Ignorance: A History of Blind Assessment and Placebo Controls in Medicine." *Bulletin of the History of Medicine* 72.3 (1998): 389–433.

———. Letter in response to Shlay et al. *Journal of the American Medical Association* 281.14 (1999): 1270.

———. "The Placebo Effect in Alternative Medicine: Can the Performance of a Healing Ritual Have Clinical Significance?" *Annals of Internal Medicine* 136.11 (2002): 817–25.

———. "Powerful Placebo: The Dark Side of the Randomised Controlled Trial." *Lancet* 351.9117 (1998): 1722–25.

Kaptchuk, Ted, and David Eisenberg. "Chiropractic: Origins, Controversies, and Contributions." *Archives of Internal Medicine* 158.20 (1998): 2215–24.

———. "The Persuasive Appeal of Alternative Medicine." *Annals of Internal Medicine* 129.12 (1998): 1061–65.

Kaptchuk, Ted, David Eisenberg, and Anthony Komaroff. "Finding Out What Works." *Newsweek* 2 Dec. 2002: 73.

————. "Pondering the Placebo Effect." *Newsweek* 2 Dec. 2002: 71.

Kaptchuk, Ted, and Catherine E. Kerr. "Unbiased Divination, Unbiased Evidence, and the Patulin Clinical Trial." *International Journal of Epidemiology* 33.2 (2004): 247–51.

Kaptchuk, Ted, et al. "Components of Placebo Effect: Randomised Controlled Trial in Patients with Irritable Bowel Syndrome." *British Medical Journal* 336.7651 (2008): 999–1003.

Kaptchuk, Ted, et al. "'Maybe I Made Up the Whole Thing': Placebos and Patients' Experiences in a Randomized Controlled Trial." *Culture, Medicine, and Psychiatry* 33.3 (2009): 382–411.

Kay, Jonathan. "Ontario Shouldn't Be Legitimizing Naturopathic 'Medicine.'" *National Post* 26 Feb. 2014. Web. 23 Mar. 2014.

Keating, Jr., Joseph C. "Philosophy in Chiropractic." *Principles and Practice of Chiropractic*. Ed. Scott Haldeman. Whitby: McGraw-Hill, 2004. 77–97.

Kelner, Merrijoy. "The Therapeutic Relationship Under Fire." *Complementary and Alternative Medicine: Challenge and Change*. Eds. Merrijoy Kelner and Beverly Wellman. New York: Routledge, 2003. 79–97.

Keränen, Lisa. *Scientific Characters: Rhetoric, Politics, and Trust in Breast Cancer Research*. Tuscaloosa: U of Alabama P, 2010.

Kidd, Joseph. "The Last Illness of Lord Beaconsfield." *Nineteenth Century* 26 (1889): 65–71.

Klass, Perri. "Learning the Language." *A Not Entirely Benign Procedure*. New York: Plume, 1987. 73–77.

Kleinman, Arthur. *The Illness Narratives: Suffering, Healing, and the Human Condition*. New York: Basic, 1988.

Klingbeil, Kurt. "Stop Bill C-51: Petition." Thepetitionsite.com. 2008. Web. 10 Sept. 2008.

Koerber, Amy. *Breast or Bottle: Contemporary Controversies in Infant-Feeding Policy and Practice*. Columbia: U South Carolina P, 2013.

Koo, John, and Sumaira Arain. "Traditional Chinese Medicine for the Treatment of Dermatologic Disorders." *Archives of Dermatology* 134.11 (1998): 1388–93.

Kopelson, Karen. "Risky Appeals: Recruiting to the Environmental Breast Cancer Movement in the Age of 'Pink Fatigue.'" *Rhetoric Society Quarterly* 43.2 (2013): 107–33.

Knoll, Elizabeth. "The Communities of Scientists and Journal Peer Review." *Journal of the American Medical Association* 263.10 (1990): 1330–32.

Knorr Cetina, Karin. *The Manufacture of Knowledge: An Essay on the Constructivist and Contextual Nature of Science*. Oxford: Pergamon, 1991.

Krouse, John H. "Alternative and Complementary Therapies: An Agenda for Otolaryngology." *Archives of Otolaryngology—Head and Neck Surgery* 124.11 (1998): 1199–1200.

Kuchment, Anna. "Chef! This Dish Needs Pain Relief." *Newsweek* 19 Nov. 2007: 72.

Kuhn, Thomas S. *The Structure of Scientific Revolutions*. Chicago: U of Chicago P, 1970.

LaFollette, Marcel C. *Making Science Our Own: Public Images of Science, 1910–1955*. Chicago: U of Chicago P, 1990.

Lakoff, Andrew. "The Right Patients for the Drug: Managing the Placebo Effect in Antidepressant Trials." *BioSocieties* 2.1 (2007): 57–71.

Lamas, Gervasio A., et al. "Effect of Disodium EDTA Chelation Regimen on Cardiovascular Events in Patients with Previous Myocardial Infarction: The TACT Randomized Trial." *Journal of the American Medical Association* 309.12 (2013): 1241–50.

Lamberg, Lynne. "Medical News and Perspectives: Dawn's Early Light to Twilight's Last Gleaming." *Journal of the American Medical Association* 280.18 (1998): 1556–58.

Latour, Bruno. *Science in Action*. Cambridge: Harvard UP, 1987.

Leach, Joan, and Deborah Dysart-Gale, eds. *Rhetorical Questions in Health and Medicine*. Lanham: Rowman and Littlefield, 2010.

Leff, Michael C. "Interpretation and the Art of the Rhetorical Critic." *Western Journal of Speech Communication* 44.4 (1980): 337–49.

Levinson, Stephen C. *Pragmatics*. New York: Cambridge UP, 1983.

Lewenstein, Bruce V. "Science and the Media." *Handbook of Science and Technology Studies*. Eds. Sheila Jasanoff, Gerald E. Markle, James C. Peterson, and Trevor J. Pinch. Thousand Oaks: Sage, 1995. 343–60.

Lewis, Bradley. "High Theory/Mass Markets: *Newsweek* Magazine and the Circuits of Medical Culture." *Perspectives in Biology and Medicine* 50.3 (2007): 262–78.

Li, Vincent W., et al. "Off-Label Dermatologic Therapies: Usage, Risks, and Mechanisms." *Archives of Dermatology* 134.11 (1998): 1449–54.

Lindsay, Bruce. "Randomized Controlled Trials of Socially Complex Nursing Interventions: Creating Bias and Unreliability?" *Journal of Advanced Nursing* 45.1 (2004): 84–94.

Liu, Tao. "Role of Acupuncturists in Acupuncture Treatment." *eCAM* 4.1 (2007): 3–6.

London, William M. "Newsweek Errs on 'Alternative Medicine,' Part 1." *National Council Against Health Fraud Newsletter* 26.1 (2003): 2.

———. "Newsweek Errs on 'Alternative Medicine,' Part 2." *National Council Against Health Fraud Newsletter* 26.2 (2003): 1–3.

———. "Newsweek's Misleading Report on 'Alternative Medicine.'" *Quackwatch*. n.p. 17 Oct. 2006. Web. 28 Oct. 2013.

Loxton, Daniel. "A Triumph of Astroturf? How a Consumer Protection Law May Be Defeated by a Faux Consumer Watchdog Campaign." *eSkeptic*. 28 May 2008. Web. 1 June 2008.

Lundberg, George. "Re: JAMA and Archives theme issues on CAM." Message to the author. 26 Aug. 2014. E-mail.

Lundberg, George, Marshall C. Paul, and Helga Fritz. "A Comparison of the Opinions of Experts and Reader as to What Topics a General Medical Journal (*JAMA*) Should Address." *JAMA* 280.3 (1998): 288–90.

Mackenzie, Elizabeth R., and Birgit Rakel, eds. *Complementary and Alternative Medicine for Older Adults: A Guide to Holistic Approaches to Healthy Aging*. New York: Springer, 2006.

MacPherson, Hugh, Lucy Thorpe, and Kate Thomas. "Beyond Needling—Therapeutic Processes in Acupuncture Care: A Qualitative Study Nested Within a Low-Back Pain Trial." *Journal of Alternative & Complementary Medicine* 12.9 (2006): 873–80.

Magazine Publishers of America. "Average Circulation for Top 100 ABC Magazines 2002." *Magazine.org*. Magazine Publishers of America, n.d. Web. 7 Aug. 2009.

Maguire, Steve. "Discourse and Adoption of Innovations: A Study of HIV/AIDS Treatments." *Health Care Management Review* 27.3 (2002): 74–88.

Margolin, Arthur, S. Kelly Avants, and Herbert D. Kleber. "Investigating Alternative Medicine Therapies in Randomized Controlled Trials." *Journal of the American Medical Association* 280.18 (1998): 1626–28.

Mason, Su, Philip Tovey, and Andrew F. Long. "Evaluating Complementary Medicine: Methodological Challenges of Randomised Controlled Trials." *British Medical Journal* 325.7368 (2002): 832–34.

McCormack, James P., and Peter Loewen. "Adding 'Value' to Clinical Practice Guidelines." *Canadian Family Physician* 53.8 (2007): 1326–27.

McCrindle, Brian W., Elizabeth Helden, and William T. Conner. "Garlic Extract Therapy in

Children with Hypercholesterolemia." *Archives of Pediatric Adolescent Medicine* 152.11 (1998): 1089–94.

McNely, Brian, Clay Spinuzzi, and Christa Teston. "Contemporary Research Methodologies in Technical Communication." *Technical Communication Quarterly* 24.1 (2015): 1–13.

Medawar, Peter. "Is the Scientific Paper Fraudulent? Yes; It Misrepresents Scientific Thought." *Saturday Review* (1964): 42–43.

Medical Research Council. *A Framework for Development and Evaluation of RCTs for Complex Interventions to Improve Health*. London, Medical Research Council: 2000.

Megill, Allan. "Introduction: Four Senses of Objectivity." *Rethinking Objectivity*. Ed. Allan Megill. Durham: Duke UP, 1994. 1–20.

Melchart, Dieter, et al. "Echinacea Root Extracts for the Prevention of Upper Respiratory Tract Infections: A Double-Blind, Placebo-Controlled Randomized Trial." *Archives of Family Medicine* 7.6 (1998): 541–45.

Mellor, Felicity. "Between Fact and Fiction: Demarcating Science from Non-Science in Popular Physics Books." *Social Studies of Science* 33.4 (2003): 509–38.

Meryn, Siegfried. "Improving Doctor-Patient Communication: Not an Option, but a Necessity." *British Medical Journal* 316.7149 (1998): 1922.

Michaels, David. *Doubt is Their Product: How Industry's Assault on Science Threatens Your Health*. New York: Oxford UP, 2008.

Michelle, Carolyn. "Media(ted) Fabrications: How the Science-Media Symbiosis Helped 'Sell' Cord Banking." *Communication & Medicine* 3.1 (2006): 55–68.

Miller, Carolyn R. "Genre as Social Action." *Quarterly Journal of Speech* 70 (1984): 151–67.

———. "Novelty and Heresy in the Debate on Nonthermal Effects of Electromagnetic Fields." *Rhetoric and Incommensurability*. Ed. Randy Allen Harris. West Lafayette: Parlor, 2005. 464–505.

Miller, Craig. "Natural Mood Remedies." *Newsweek* 2 Dec. 2002: 70.

Mishler, Elliot G. *The Discourse of Medicine: Dialectics of Medical Interviews*. Norwood: Ablex, 1984.

Mitka, Mike. "FDA Never Promised an Herb Garden—But Sellers and Buyers Eager to See One Grow." *Journal of the American Medical Association* 280.18 (1998): 1554–56.

Moirand, Sophie. "Communicative and Cognitive Dimensions of Discourse on Science in the French Mass Media." *Discourse Studies* 5.2 (2003): 175–206.

Mol, Annemarie. *The Logic of Care: Health and the Problem of Patient Choice*. New York: Routledge, 2008.

Morreim, E. Haavi. "A Dose of Our Own Medicine: Alternative Medicine, Conventional Medicine, and the Standards of Science." *Journal of Law, Medicine, and Ethics* 31.2 (2003): 222–35.

Mudry, Jessica. *Measured Meals: Nutrition in America*. Albany: SUNY P, 2009.

Mulkay, Michael, and G. Nigel Gilbert. "Replication and Mere Replication." *Philosophy of the Social Sciences* 16.1 (1986): 21–37.

Murray, T. J. "Why the Medical Humanities?" *Dalhousie Medical Journal* 26.1 (1998): 46–50.

Myers, Greg. "Discourse Studies of Scientific Popularization: Questioning the Boundaries." *Discourse Studies* 5.2 (2003): 265–79.

———. *Writing Biology*. Madison: U of Wisconsin P, 1990.

Mykhalovskiy, Eric, and Lorna Weir. "The Problem of Evidence-Based Medicine: Directions for Social Science." *Social Science & Medicine* 59.5 (2004): 1059–69.

Nagel, Thomas. *The View from Nowhere*. New York: Oxford UP, 1986.

Nahin, Richard L., et al. "Costs of Complementary and Alternative Medicine (CAM) and Frequency of Visits to CAM Practitioners: United States, 2007." *National Health Statistics Reports* 18 (2009): 1–14.

Nahin, Richard L., and Stephen E. Straus. "Research into Complementary and Alternative Medicine: Problems and Potential." *British Medical Journal* 322.7279 (2001): 161–64.

National Center for Complementary and Alternative Medicine. "CAM Basics: What Is CAM?" *National Center for Complementary and Alternative Medicine.* National Institutes of Health, Feb. 2007. Web. Aug. 22 2009.

Nelkin, Dorothy. *Selling Science: How the Press Covers Science and Technology.* New York: Freeman, 1995.

"Newsweek Examines Back Pain." *Dynamic Chiropractic* 22.11 (2004): n.p.

"Newsweek Validates Complementary and Alternative Therapies for Back Pain." *Massage Today* 4.6 (2004): n.p.

Nichter, Mark, and Jennifer Thompson. "For My Wellness, Not Just My Illness: North Americans' Use of Dietary Supplements." *Culture, Medicine & Psychiatry* 30.2 (2006): 175–222.

"NIH Consensus Conference on Acupuncture." *Journal of the American Medical Association* 280.17 (1998): 1518–24.

Nisly, Nicole L., et al. "Dietary Supplement Polypharmacy: An Unrecognized Public Health Problem?" *eCAM* 5 Dec. 2007. Web. 8 June 2008.

Nissen, Steven E. "Concerns about Reliability in the Trial to Assess Chelation Therapy (TACT)." *Journal of the American Medical Association* 309. 12 (2013): 1293–94.

Noonan, David. "For the Littlest Patients." *Newsweek* 2 Dec. 2002: 58.

O'Connor, Mary E., et al. "Relaxation Training and Breast Milk Secretory IgA." *Archives of Pediatric Adolescent Medicine* 152.11 (1998): 1065–70.

Odell, Lee, Dixie Goswami, and Anne Herrington. "The Discourse-Based Interview: A Procedure for Exploring the Tacit Knowledge of Writers in Nonacademic Settings." *Writing in Nonacademic Settings.* Eds. Lee Odell and Dixie Goswami. New York: Guilford, 1985. 221–36.

O'Hara, MaryAnn, et al. "A Review of 12 Commonly Used Medicinal Herbs." *Archives of Family Medicine* 7.6 (1998): 523–36.

Olivieri, Nancy F., et al. "Long-Term Safety and Effectiveness of Iron-Chelation Therapy with Deferiprone for Thalassemia Major." *New England Journal of Medicine* 339.7 (1998): 417–23.

Ong, L. M. L., et al. "Doctor-Patient Communication: A Review of the Literature." *Social Science & Medicine* 40.7 (1995): 903–18.

Oreskes, Naomi, and Erik M. Conway. *Merchants of Doubt: How a Handful of Scientists Obscured the Truth on Issues from Tobacco Smoke to Global Warming.* New York: Bloomsbury, 2011.

Organ, Claude H., Jr. "Alternative Medicine and Surgery." *Archives of Surgery* 133.11 (1998): 1153–54.

O'Sullivan, Richard L., Graeme Lipper, and Ethan A. Lerner. "The Neuro-Immuno-Cutaneous-Endocrine Network: Relationship of Mind and Skin." *Archives of Dermatology* 134.11 (1998): 1431–35.

Oths, Kathryn. "Communication in a Chiropractic Clinic: How a D. C. Treats His Patients." *Culture, Medicine, and Psychiatry* 18.1 (1994): 83–113.

———. "Unintended Therapy: Psychotherapeutic Aspects of Chiropractic." *Ethnopsychiatry: The Cultural Construction of Professional and Folk Psychiatries.* Ed. Atwood D. Gaines. New York: SUNY P, 1992. 85–123.

Oumeish, Oumeish Youssef. "The Philosophical, Cultural, and Historical Aspects of Complementary, Alternative, Unconventional, and Integrative Medicine in the Old World." *Archives of Dermatology* 134.11 (1998): 1373–86.

Palmer, Mary E., et al. "Adverse Events Associated with Dietary Supplements: An Observational Study." *Lancet* 361.9352 (2003): 101–06.

Pappas, Sam, and Adam Perlman. "Complementary and Alternative Medicine: The Importance of Doctor-Patient Communication." *Medical Clinics of North America* 86.1 (2002): 1–10.

Paré, Anthony. "Genre and Identity: Individuals, Institutions, and Ideology." *The Rhetoric and Ideology of Genre*. Eds. Richard Coe, Lorelei Lingard, and Tatiana Teslenko. Cresskill: Hampton, 2002. 57–71.

Park, Robert L. *Voodoo Science: The Road from Foolishness to Fraud*. New York: Oxford UP, 2000.

———. "What's New: Friday, November 29, 2002." *What's New by Bob Park*. University of Maryland. 29 Nov. 2002. Web. 20 May 2009.

Paterson, Charlotte, and Paul Dieppe. "Characteristic and Incidental (Placebo) Effects in Complex Interventions such as Acupuncture." *British Medical Journal* 330.7501 (2005): 1202–05.

Paul, Danette. "Spreading Chaos: The Role of Popularizations in the Diffusion of Scientific Ideas." *Written Communication* 21.1 (2004): 32–68.

Paul, Danette, Davida Charney, and Aimee Kendall. "Moving Beyond the Moment: Reception Studies in the Rhetoric of Science." *Journal of Business and Technical Communication* 15.3 (2001): 372–98.

Peabody, Francis W. "The Care of the Patient." *Journal of the American Medical Association* 88 (1927): 877–82.

Perelman, Chaim. *The Realm of Rhetoric*. Notre Dame: U of Notre Dame P, 1982.

Perry, Angela. *American Medical Association Guide to Talking to Your Doctor*. New York: Wiley, 2001.

Petryna, Adriana. "Clinical Trials Offshored: On Private Sector Science and Public Health." *BioSocieties* 2.1 (2007): 21–40.

Pezzullo, Phaedra. "Resisting 'National Breast Cancer Awareness Month': The Rhetoric of Counter-Publics and their Cultural Performances." *Quarterly Journal of Speech* 89.4 (2003): 345–65.

Popper, Karl. *The Logic of Scientific Discovery*. New York: Routledge, 2002.

Porter, Roy. *Quacks: Fakers and Charlatans in English Medicine*. Charleston: Tempus, 2000.

Porter, Sam. "The Patient and Power: Sociological Perspectives on the Consequences of Holistic Care." *Health and Social Care in the Community* 5.1 (1997): 17–20.

Porter, Theodore. *Trust in Numbers: The Pursuit of Objectivity in Science and Public Life*. Princeton: Princeton UP, 1995.

Prelli, Lawrence J. "Rhetorical Logic and the Integration of Rhetoric and Science." *Communication Monographs* 57 (1990): 315–22.

———. *A Rhetoric of Science: Inventing Scientific Discourse*. Columbia: U of South Carolina P, 1989.

Prince, Ellen. "Toward a Taxonomy of Given-New Information." *Radical Pragmatics*. Ed. Peter Cole. New York: Academic, 1981. 223–55.

Reardon, Thomas R. Preface. *Alternative Medicine: An Objective Assessment*. Ed. Phil B. Fontanarosa. Chicago: American Medical Association, 2000. v.

Reiser, Stanley Joel. *Medicine and the Reign of Technology*. New York: Cambridge UP, 1978.

Renckens, C. N. M. "Alternative Treatments in Reproductive Medicine: Much Ado about Nothing." *Human Reproduction* 17.3 (2002): 528–33.

Rennie, Drummond. "Fourth International Congress on Peer Review in Biomedical Publica-
    tion." *Journal of the American Medical Association* 287.21 (2002): 2759–60.

"Research." *Program in Placebo Studies & Therapeutic Encounter (PiPS).* Program in Placebo
    Studies & Therapeutic Encounter (PiPS), n.d. Web. 30 June 2015.

Richard, Dan. "What Counts As Evidence? A Personal Odyssey into Alternative Care." *Archives
    of Family Medicine* 7.6 (1998): 598–99.

Richards, Evelleen. *Vitamin C and Cancer: Medicine or Politics?* London: Macmillan, 1991.

Ritenbaugh, Cheryl K. "Developing Patient-Centered Measures for Outcomes of CAM Thera-
    pies [Grant1R01AT003314–01A1]." National Center for Complementary and Alternative
    Medicine. National Institutes of Health. 27 May 2009. Web. 1 June 2009.

Ruggie, Mary. *Marginal to Mainstream: Alternative Medicine in America.* New York: Cambridge
    UP, 2004.

Sackett, David L., William M. C. Rosenberg, J. A. Muir Gray, R. Brian Haynes, and W. Scott
    Richardson. "Evidence Based Medicine: What it Is and What it Isn't." *British Medical Journal*
    312.7023 (1996): 71–72.

Sain, Abd Hamid Mat. "Evidence-Based Medicine Revisited." Letter in response to Sackett et al.
    British Medical Journal (26 Jan. 2004): n.p. Web. 26 June 2009.

Saks, Mike. *Orthodox and Alternative Medicine: Politics, Professionalization, and Health Care.*
    London: Continuum, 2003.

Schryer, Catherine F. "The Lab vs. the Clinic: Sites of Competing Genres." *Genre and the New
    Rhetoric.* Eds. Aviva Freedman and Peter Medway. London: Taylor and Francis, 1995. 105–24.

Schryer, Catherine F., and Philippa Spoel. "Genre Theory, Health-Care Discourse, and Profes-
    sional Identity Formation." *Journal of Business and Technical Communication* 19.3 (2005):
    249–78.

Schuster, Mary M. Lay. [Mary M. Lay.] *The Rhetoric of Midwifery: Gender, Knowledge, and
    Power.* New Brunswick: Rutgers UP, 2000.

Schwartz, Lisa M., Steven Woloshin, and Linda Baczek. "Media Coverage of Scientific Meetings:
    Too Much, Too Soon?" *Journal of the American Medical Association* 287.21 (2002): 2859–63.

"The Science of Cooking." *Evidence-Based Living.* Cornell University, n.d. Web. 5 July 2015.

Scott, J. Blake. "Extending Rhetorical-Cultural Analysis: Transformations of Home HIV Test-
    ing." *College English* 65.4 (2003): 349–69.

———. *Risky Rhetoric: AIDS and the Cultural Practices of HIV Testing.* Carbondale: Southern
    Illinois UP, 2003.

Segal, Judy Z. "Breast Cancer Narratives as Public Rhetoric: Genre Itself and the Maintenance of
    Ignorance." *Linguistics and the Human Sciences* 3.1 (2008): 3–23.

———. "'Compliance' to 'Concordance': A Critical View." *Journal of Medical Humanities* 28.2
    (2007): 81–96.

———. "'Female Sexual Dysfunction' and a Rhetoric of Values." *Rhetoric of Healthcare: Essays
    Toward a New Disciplinary Inquiry.* Eds. Barbara Heifferon and Stuart C. Brown. Cresskill:
    Hampton, 2008. 33–50.

———. *Health and the Rhetoric of Medicine.* Carbondale: Southern Illinois UP, 2005.

———. "Illness as Argumentation: A Prolegomenon to the Rhetorical Study of Contestable
    Complaints." *health: An Interdisciplinary Journal for the Social Study of Health, Illness, and
    Medicine* 11.2 (2007): 227–44.

———. "Interdisciplinarity and Bibliography in Rhetoric of Health and Medicine." *Technical
    Communication Quarterly* 14.3 (2005): 311–18.

———. "Internet Health and the Twenty-First Century Patient: A Rhetorical View." *Written Communication* 26.4 (2009): 351–69.

———. "Rhetoric of Health and Medicine." *The Sage Handbook of Rhetorical Studies*. Eds. Andrea Lunsford, Kirt H. Wilson, and Rosa A. Eberly. Thousand Oaks: Sage, 2009. 227–46.

———. "The Sexualization of the Medical." *Journal of Sex Research* 49.4 (2012): 369–78.

———. "Strategies of Influence in Medical Authorship." *Social Science & Medicine* 37.4 (1993): 521–30.

Seigel, Marika. *The Rhetoric of Pregnancy*. Chicago: U Chicago P, 2013.

Shang, Charles. "The Future of Integrative Medicine." *Archives of Internal Medicine* 161.4 (2001): 613–14.

Shlay, Judith C., Kathryn Shaloner, Mitchell B. Max, Bob Flaws, Patricia Reichelderfer, Deborah Wentworth, Shauna Hillman, et al. "Acupuncture and Amitriptyline for Pain Due to HIV-Related Peripheral Neuropathy: A Randomized Controlled Trial." *Journal of the American Medical Association* 280.18 (1998): 1590–95.

Shmerling, Robert, Catherine Ulbricht, and Ethan Basch. "Options for Arthritis Pain." *Newsweek* 2 Dec. 2002: 53.

Simons, Herbert W. "The Rhetoric of the Scientific Research Report: 'Drug-pushing' in a Medical Journal Article." *The Recovery of Rhetoric: Persuasive Discourse and Disciplinarity in the Human Sciences*. Eds. R. H. Roberts and J. M. Good. Charlottesville: UP of Virginia, 1993. 148–64.

Singh, Simon, and Edzard Ernst. *Trick or Treatment: The Undeniable Facts about Alternative Medicine*. New York: Norton, 2008.

Smolle, Josef, Gerhard Prause, and Helmut Kerl. "A Double-Blind, Controlled Clinical Trial of Homeopathy and an Analysis of Lunar Phases and Postoperative Outcome." *Archives of Dermatology* 134.11 (1998): 1368–70.

Solomon, Martha. "The Rhetoric of Dehumanization: An Analysis of Medical Reports of the Tuskeegee Syphilis Project." *Western Journal of Speech Communication* 49.4 (1985): 233–47.

Solomon, Miriam. "Epistemological Reflections on the Art of Medicine and Narrative Medicine." *Perspectives in Biology and Medicine* 51.3 (2008): 406–17.

Spafford, Marlee, et al. "Accessibility and Order: Crossing Borders in Child Abuse Forensic Reports." *Technical Communication Quarterly* 19.2 (2010): 118–43.

Span, Paula. "Fighting Words Are Rarer Among British Doctors." *New York Times International* 22 Apr. 2014. Web. 16 Nov. 2014.

"Special Report: Health for Life: Inside the Science of Alternative Medicine." [Title page.] *Newsweek* 2 Dec. 2002: 45.

Spoel, Philippa. "Communicating Values, Valuing Community through Health-Care Websites: Midwifery's Online Ethos and Public Communication in Ontario." *Technical Communication Quarterly* 17.3 (2008): 264–88.

———. "Midwifery, Consumerism, and the Ethics of Informed Choice." *Bordering Biomedicine*. Eds. Vera Kalitzkus and Peter L. Twohig. New York: Rodopi, 2006. 197–213.

Spoel, Philippa, and Susan James. "The Textual Standardization of Midwives' Professional Relationships." *Technostyle* 19.1 (2003): 3–29.

Star, Susan Leigh, and Geoffrey C. Bowker. "Enacting Silence: Residual Categories as a Challenge for Ethics, Information Systems, and Communication." *Ethics and Information Technology* 9.4 (2007): 273–80.

Star, Susan Leigh, and James R. Griesemer. "Institutional Ecology, 'Translations,' and Boundary

Objects: Amateurs and Professionals in Berkeley's Museum of Vertebrate Zoology, 1907–39." *Social Studies of Science* 19.3 (1989): 387–420.

Starr, Paul. *The Social Transformation of American Medicine*. New York: Basic, 1982.

Stein, Howard F. *American Medicine as Culture*. San Francisco: Westfield, 1990.

Stener-Victorin, Elisabet, et al. "Alternative Treatments in Reproductive Medicine: Much Ado About Nothing: Acupuncture—A Method of Treatment in Reproductive Medicine: Lack of Evidence of an Effect Does Not Equal Evidence of The Lack of an Effect." *Human Reproduction* 17.8 (2002): 1942–46.

Stewart, Moira. "Towards a Global Definition of Patient Centered Care." *British Medical Journal* 322.7284 (2001): 444–45.

Stewart, Moira, and Judith Belle Brown. "Patient-Centredness in Medicine." *Evidence-Based Patient Choice: Inevitable or Impossible*. Eds. Adrian Edwards and Glyn Elwyn. New York: Oxford UP, 2001. 97–117.

Stewart, Moira, and Debra Roter, eds. *Communicating with Medical Patients*. Newbury Park: Sage, 1989.

Stillar, Glenn. *Analyzing Everyday Texts: Discourse, Rhetoric, and Social Perspectives*. Thousand Oaks: Sage, 1998.

Stop C-51: The Official Stop C-51 Website. Truehope, n.d. Web. 2008. 1 June 2008.

Strauss, Stephen. "Can't We Find a Better Name for the Placebo Effect?" *CBC.ca* 16 Mar. 2007. Canadian Broadcasting Corporation. Web. 17 Jan. 2008.

Sugarman, Jeremy, and Larry Burk. "Physicians' Ethical Obligations Regarding Alternative Medicine." *Journal of the American Medical Association* 280.18 (1998): 1623–25.

Sullivan, Dale L. "Keeping the Rhetoric Orthodox: Forum Control in Science." *Technical Communication Quarterly* 9.2 (2000): 125–46.

Swales, John. *Genre Analysis: English in Academic and Research Settings*. New York: Cambridge UP, 1990.

Swenson, Sara L., et al. "Patient-Centered Communication: Do Patients Really Prefer It?" *Journal of General Internal Medicine* 19.11 (2004): 1069–79.

Taubes, Gary. "Do We Really Know What Makes Us Healthy?" *New York Times Magazine* 16 Sept. 2007. Web. 10 Oct. 2007.

Tausk, Francisco A. "Alternative Medicine: Is It All in Your Mind?" *Archives of Dermatology* 134.11 (1998): 1422–25.

Taylor, Charles Alan. *Defining Science: A Rhetoric of Demarcation*. Madison: U of Wisconsin P, 1996.

Theodoropoulos, Demetrios. "Professional Identity and its Responsibilities." *Archives of Pediatric & Adolescent Medicine* 152.6 (1998): 606.

———. Reply to letter of Gerald Ente. *Archives of Pediatric & Adolescent Medicine* 152.11 (1998): 1154.

Thomsen, Robert J. "Spirituality in Medical Practice." *Archives of Dermatology* 134.11 (1998): 1443–46.

"Top of the Week." *Newsweek* 2 Dec. 2002: 3.

Ulett, George A. Letter in response to Shlay et al. *Journal of the American Medical Association* 281.14 (1999): 1270–71.

Underwood, Anne. "Learning From China." *Newsweek* 2 Dec. 2002: 54.

———. "The Magic of Mushrooms." *Newsweek* 3 Nov. 2003: 61.

van Weel, Chris, and J. Andre Knottnerus. "Evidence-Based Interventions and Comprehensive Treatment." *Lancet* 353.9156 (1999): 916–18.

Vickers, Andrew. "Message to Complementary and Alternative Medicine: Evidence Is a Better Friend Than Power." *BMC Complementary and Alternative Medicine* 1.1 (2001): n.p. Web. 20 Aug 2009.

Viens, Adrian M., and Julian Savulescu. "Introduction to the Olivieri Symposium." *Journal of Medical Ethics* 30 (2004): 1–7.

Villanueva-Russell, Yvonne. "Evidence-Based Medicine and Its Implications for the Profession of Chiropractic." *Social Science & Medicine* 60.3 (2005): 545–61.

Vincent, C., and A. Furnham. "Why Do Patients Turn to Complementary Medicine? An Empirical Study." *British Journal of Clinical Psychology* 35 (1996): 37–48.

Wagner, Edward H., et al. "Finding Common Ground: Patient-Centeredness and Evidence-Based Chronic Illness Care." *Journal of Alternative and Complementary Medicine* 11 Suppl. 1 (2005): S7–S15.

Wahlberg, Ayo. "A Quackery with a Difference: New Medical Pluralism and the Problem of 'Dangerous Practitioners' in the United Kingdom." *Social Science & Medicine* 65.11 (2007): 2307–16.

Wahlberg, Ayo, and Linsey McGoey. "An Elusive Evidence Base: The Construction and Governance of Randomized Controlled Trials." *BioSocieties* 2.1 (2007): 1–10.

Weaver, Richard M. "Concealed Rhetoric in Scientistic Sociology." *Language Is Sermonic: Richard M. Weaver on the Nature of Rhetoric.* Eds. Richard L. Johannesen, Rennard Strickland, and Ralph T. Eubanks. Baton Rouge: Louisiana State UP, 1970. 139–58.

Weiger, Wendy, and David Eisenberg. "Easing the Treatment." *Newsweek* 2 Dec. 2002: 49.

"Weighing Alternatives." *Newsweek* Spring/Summer 1999: 61.

Weigold, Michael F. "Communicating Science: A Review of the Literature." *Science Communication* 23.2 (2001): 164–93.

Weisz, George. "From Clinical Counting to Evidence-Based Medicine." *Body Counts: Medical Quantification in Historical and Sociological Perspective.* Eds. Gérard Jorland, George Weisz, and Annick Opinel. Montréal: McGill-Queen's UP, 2005. 377–93.

Wessely, Simon. "A Defence of the Randomized Controlled Trial in Mental Health." *BioSocieties* 2.1 (2007): 115–27.

White, Adrian R., Karl-Ludwig Resch, and Edzard Ernst. "Randomized Trial of Acupuncture for Nicotine Withdrawal Symptoms." *Archives of Internal Medicine* 158.20 (1998): 2251–55.

Whorton, James C. "From Cultism to CAM: The Flexner Report Revisited." *Complementary Health Practice Review* 6.2 (2001): 113–25.

———. *Nature Cures: The History of Alternative Medicine in America.* New York: Oxford UP, 2002.

Will, Catherine M. "The Alchemy of Clinical Trials." *BioSocieties* 2.1 (2007): 85–99.

Willerton, Russell. "Visual Metonymy and Synecdoche: Rhetoric for Stage-Setting Images." *Journal of Technical Writing & Communication* 35.1 (2005): 3–31.

Wilson, Greg, and Carl G. Herndl. "Boundary Objects as Rhetorical Exigence: Knowledge Mapping and Interdisciplinary Cooperation at the Los Alamos National Laboratory." *Journal of Business and Technical Communication* 21.2 (2007): 129–54.

Wolff, Nancy. "Using Randomized Controlled Trials to Evaluate Socially Complex Services: Problems, Challenges and Recommendations." *Journal of Mental Health Policy and Economics* 3.2 (2000): 97–109.

Wolpe, Paul Root. "Medical Culture and CAM Culture: Science and Ritual in the Academic Medical Center." *The Role of Complementary and Alternative Medicine: Accommodating Pluralism.* Ed. Daniel Callahan. Washington, DC: Georgetown UP, 2002. 163–71.

Wong, Albert H. C., Michael Smith, and Heather S. Boon. "Herbal Remedies in Psychiatric Practice." *Archives of General Psychiatry* 55.11 (1998): 1033–44.

Writing Group for the Women's Health Initiative Investigators. "Risks and Benefits of Estrogen Plus Progestin in Healthy Postmenopausal Women: Principal Results from the Women's Health Initiative Randomized Controlled Trial." *Journal of the American Medical Association* 288.3 (2002): 321–33.

Yeo, Richard R. "Scientific Method and the Rhetoric of Science in Britain, 1830–1917." *The Politics and Rhetoric of Scientific Method.* Eds. John A. Schuster and Richard A. Yeo. Boston: D. Reidel, 1986. 259–97.

Index